HEALTHY EATING MANIFESTO

Linda Celauro

HEALTHY EATING MANIFESTO

Weigh Less ~ Savour More

Linda Celauro

DEDICATION

Lovingly dedicated to my husband, Nathan, whose
boundless energy leaves me speechless!
My lovely daughter, Lauren Rossi, who inspires me
everyday. She has totally embraced a holistic lifestyle
and has authored healthy eating publications.
To my extended family and friends, who without your
input, none of this would be possible.

CONTENTS

Acknowledgements

This one's for you. That's right.
If it's okay with you,
I'd like to say a more public thank you.
You deserve to be acknowledged.

Special thanks to:
Joshua Rosenthal, Founder and Director of
Institute for Integrative Nutrition
and Lindsey Smith for their guidance
in getting the book of my dreams
out into the world.

For those of you who know me, you know who you
are; I want to thank you for putting up with me
when I got uber-stressed.

INTRODUCTION

Do you LOVE the good-life?

Ready to kick up your heels and party at a moment's notice?

Comfortable in flip-flops or stilettos?

Jeans or Black-Tie?

Have you recently noticed those jeans do not fit quite the way they used to?

You probably know what to do; maybe you even have a Ph.D. in dieting?

You're savvy, sophisticated and LOVE to live life to the fullest.

So—what's eating you?

Despite all of your efforts, do you still need to shed a few pounds?

Been there and done that....

Say No More,

I HEAR YOU LOUD AND CLEAR!

I decided to write this book for two reasons.
The first reason is:
The plain and simple fact is that most diets *fail*.

Many people want to lose weight to improve their health and their appearance. There are way too many commercial weight loss programs on the market; most are expensive, capitalizing on the tremendous demand.
Of those programs, many are ineffective.
There is no magic potion, pill or program. Don't be sucked in by empty promises or ridiculous claims of miraculous results.

Each year millions of Americans and people from all over the world enroll in commercial and self-help weight loss programs. Healthcare providers know little about these programs because of the absence of systematic reviews. Many of the existing studies present the best-case scenario because they do not account for people who drop out of the program. Unfortunately, many patients and their doctors know little about the effectiveness and safety of these programs, either. In the short term, results may be attainable but long term results are doubtful.

The old-fashioned myth of calorie counting and deprivation does not make for a healthy weight loss plan.

Aren't you just sick and tired of buying book after book, trying diet after diet, and still not experiencing the changes you want and desire?

The second reason is:

Most of us love to have a good time, and that includes "party-time."

So, if you are anything like me, then you:

* are totally in Love with Fine-Dining almost to a fault.
* like to travel where the best of intentions can turn to Sh*T!
* love to laugh to the point of tears with your best friends over a bottle of wine.

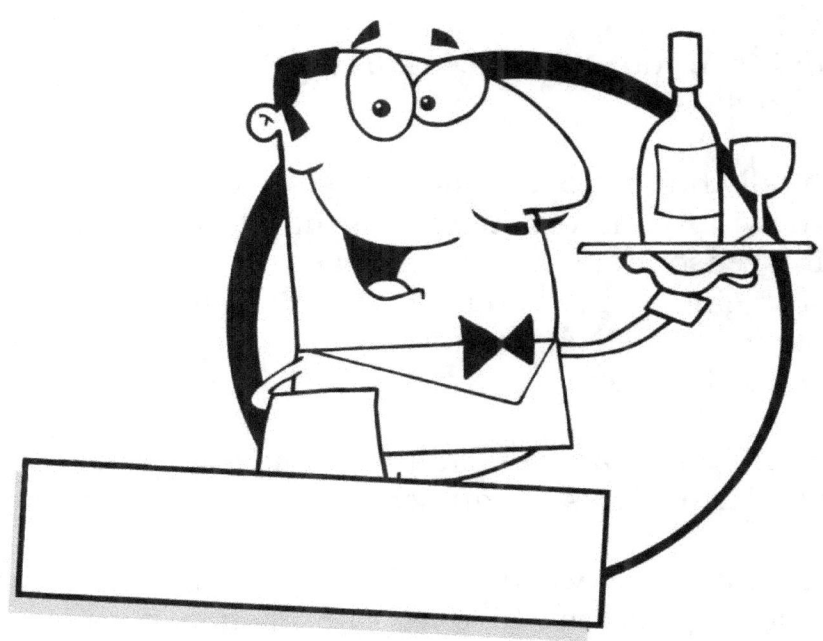

Imagine freeing yourself from the "diet mentality" and *not* feeling guilty about breaking the rules.

Haven't you felt like screaming at all those "psycho" perfectionists out there anyway?

I'm a firm believer that life is all about the yin and yang.
I strive to find the balance that keeps me happy, healthy, fit and trim.
While at the same time, not skipping a beat when it comes to having a good time.

Well, I have good news for you: I'm here to help, and you do NOT need to overhaul your entire lifestyle.

Small changes over time = huge rewards.
Knowing your unique eating habits can help you find reasonable ways to change.
Changing your behavior and letting go of old-fashioned beliefs are key to long-term, successful weight loss and vibrant health.

In this fast-paced, media-overloaded world, it's no wonder we are so confused about eating properly.

As children, we were somehow "tricked" into believing food can be used to punish or reward.

As a young child, did you ever hear?

"If you don't finish what's on your plate, you'll be sent to your room."
"You can have dessert, but only if you eat your vegetables first."
"If you behave, I'll take you out for ice cream."

Hello! Food should not be used to punish or pacify, but to satisfy.

It's time to take matters into our own hands and "unlearn" this BS.

Life is short - let's make the best of it together.

What will it take to stop focusing on food and weight and start focusing on *loving life?*

Healthy
is the
New Sexy

CHAPTER 1

FOOD - The "Other" F-Word

Once upon a time, we ate REAL Food.
~ The End ~

Wish it ended there......BUT,
We've come a long way *baby! (NOT in a good way)*

So what does this four-letter word really mean?

food
food/
nun
noun: **food**; plural noun: **foods**
　1.　any nutritious substance that people or
　　　animals eat or drink, or that plants absorb,
　　　in order to maintain life and growth.

Food is meant to maintain life, growth and the
health of our body.
Food is the information for our body to function
properly. If we don't get the correct information,
we are at risk for the development of diseases and
other unhealthy conditions. Simple, right?

FOOD is fuel for our body (imagine a car running on low-grade fuel)?
FOOD provides our body with essential nutrients.
FOOD allows the body to function properly.
FOOD acts to prevent disease.

"Let food be thy medicine"
~ Hippocrates

Famous last words,
"I'm going on a diet."

The phrase suggests that, like a vacation trip, there is a beginning and an end. We dream of the day we will reach our weight goal and how wonderful it will be when we don't have to lead a life of painful deprivation.

We long for the day when we no longer have to clench our teeth as we refuse a favorite dish that always causes us to salivate in our sleep. We reach for the carrot and celery sticks without anticipation or enthusiasm while torturing ourselves with visions of the special treats we will enjoy when the diet is over. In the back of our minds, there is a comforting little tape playing, promising us that when our weight loss campaign is over, we will be able to stop counting calories and depriving ourselves of the foods we love.

Uh, hello?

Allowing ourselves to think of a diet as a delineated, restricted period within our total life span is a sure avenue back to tent city (that refers to what we wear, not where we live). To have any hope of attaining permanent health and weight control, we must approach it as a lifelong effort, watching our intake day after day, week after week, year after year.

You feel your heart sinking in your chest. You think if I have to live like this all the time, it's just not worth it! That little voice promises you that you are different. You can relax because now you know how to lose weight; you can do it anytime you want. Gain five pounds, and you can go back on your diet and be back to goal in no time at all.

But you won't. Many of us still believe that once our weight is down, it will be so easy to go on a short diet if we gain back a few pounds. It doesn't work that way, though, does it? We start gaining a pound here and a pound there, but then there are some special events coming up and a diet would be so damn inconvenient.

We don't go back on our diet until we have gained enough weight to develop the self-disgust that warrants a new period of serious deprivation. We have become a full-fledged member of the yo-yo club, that vast majority of dieters who cannot keep the weight off for more than a few weeks.

The reasons we go on and off diets are numerous: they are boring, depressing, and very uncomfortable. They set us apart from friends, family, and coworkers who continue to snack, to feast, and to celebrate. We resent how diets make us feel and how they impact our daily lives.

Let's look at the whole picture from a different perspective for a minute.

We are not going on a diet. We are starting our diet-for-life.
While the prospect may appall you, don't say you can't do it just yet.

Can you stay on a healthy eating diet permanently? Yes, you can, because you're not restricting yourself from anything for life. Should you stay on a diet for the rest of your life? Yes, you probably should as long as you are getting a balance of foods.

If you don't know where you are going, all roads lead to nowhere.

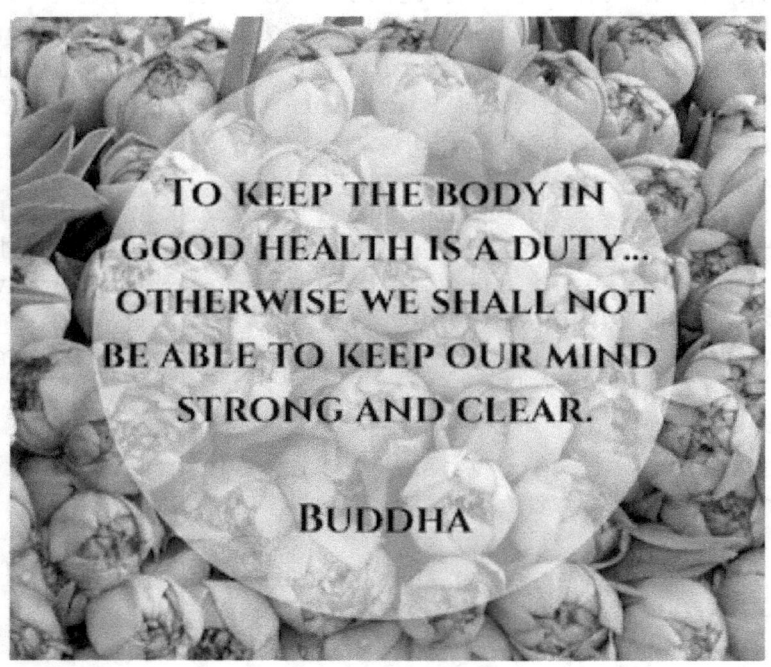

TO KEEP THE BODY IN GOOD HEALTH IS A DUTY... OTHERWISE WE SHALL NOT BE ABLE TO KEEP OUR MIND STRONG AND CLEAR.

BUDDHA

"SAD" Standard American Diet

<u>Some Scary and Startling Stats</u>

According to Yale's Rudd Center, the US fast-food chains like McDonalds, Wendy's, and Burger King spent $4.6 billion on advertising in 2012.
In contrast, the Center for Nutrition Policy and Promotion, the USDA's sub-agency that "works to improve the health and well-being of Americans by developing and promoting dietary guidance that links scientific research to the nutrition needs of consumers," had a proposed budget of $8.7 million in 2013.

I often question why do we
eat so much crap?

Considering we are one of the wealthiest nations,
why in the world are we so uninformed?

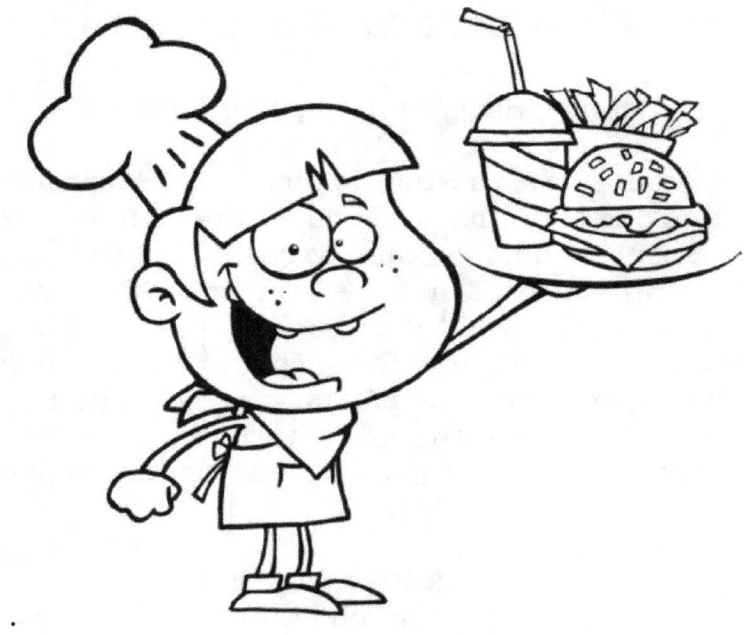

We should be more aware than ever but in the age of information, there's sadly so much misinformation out there.

According to the Organization for Economic Cooperation and Development (OECD), the United States has the highest share of health spending. Americans are fatter and sicker than people in other comparable countries; the OECD finds.

Of the 34 countries of the (OECD), the life expectancy in the United States is now lower than the average.

So, the sad fact is Americans pay more for healthcare than any other nation, yet we are far from the healthiest.

In fact, not only are we living with more chronic illness than ever, America now takes the "cake" as the most obese country in the world.
Not worthy of a celebration.

Obesity rates have doubled since 1970 according to the National Center for Health Statistics.
Over 2/3 of the American population is considered to be overweight or obese.

 REALLY? - NOT Cool

A way to calculate obesity is as follows:
Body mass index, or BMI is a common measure of body fat based on height and weight.

(Calculate your body mass index at www.webmd.com/diet/calc-bmi-plus.)

A BMI of 30 or greater is considered obese,

25-29.9 overweight

18.5-24.9 normal range

< 18.5 underweight

People who are obese are far more likely to be diagnosed with high blood pressure, high cholesterol, diabetes, or to be at greater risk for heart attack.

In addition to the major obesity problem, it is no wonder we are slipping in terms of life-expectancy.
Today's kids are now expected to live shorter lives than their parents ~ GASP!

According to the UK publication, the Daily Mail,
(compared to 222 of the world's nations)
the United States ranks #51 in terms of longevity,
just behind Guam.

Much of the weight loss industry likes to focus on
overweight Americans. That's where the money is for
them. But the truth is, much of the world is
overweight, too.
If this is not an eye-opener, I don't know what is. We
need to wake up and smell the coffee. It is clear that
we need to clean up our act and lead a healthier
lifestyle to make up for lost ground.

Knowledge is Power

EXIT EXCUSES

Leave them at the Door

Have *you* ever used any of these phrases?

— Its too much work
— Healthy food costs too much
— I can't afford a fancy gym
or Yoga or Pilates
— I don't have enough time...
— And BLAH! BLAH! BLAH!

STOP whining already

Since when did you become NOT worth it?

My questions to you:

Have you ever taken a vacation that was a real stretch to your budget?
Bought yourself something a bit too extravagant just because you had to have it, and you knew you shouldn't have?
Bought something for yourself that you were embarrassed to tell your spouse or significant other?

If you are human, your answer is yes.

I always say, it's a matter of pay me now or pay me later.

Why wouldn't you want to look good and feel great?

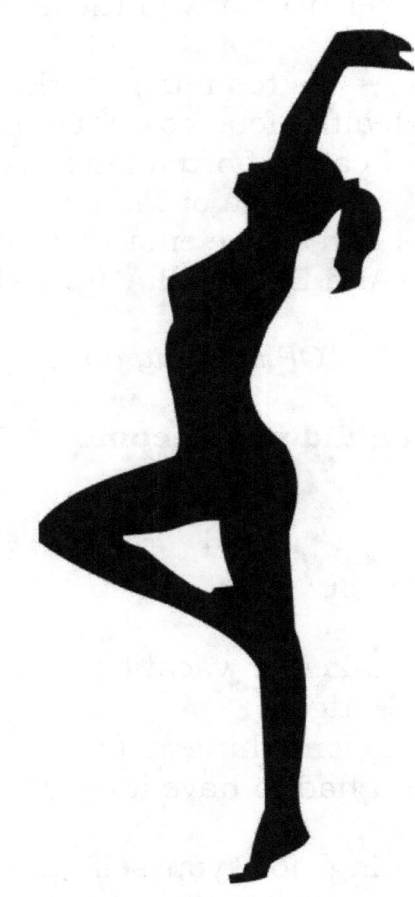

You ARE so worth it!

Invest in your health now, so you don't have to pay for it later.

Are you ready to?
Replace those mushy, high starch meals with real whole fresh foods?
Improve your health, increase energy, and watch your tummy fade?
Discard the concept of going on a diet and embrace a lifelong healthy eating plan that leaves you in control for the rest of your healthy, slender and *amazing* life?

What you eat plays arguably the most important role on your overall health and wellness. Thus, proper diet should be the most important factor of any and every health seeker.

Let's learn how to improve your health and weight loss goals by introducing several healthy habits that are easy to integrate into your current lifestyle.

"Everything in excess is opposed to nature."
~ Hippocrates

CHAPTER 2
Get Smart: The ABC's of Vitamins and Minerals

Vitamins and minerals are often called micronutrients. Your body only requires tiny amounts of them. Failing to get even those small quantities can cause disease.

What are vitamins, and why do they have such an important role in our lives?
What are these nutrients that your body so craves and what do they do to keep you healthy?
How can you get these vitamins and how are they best absorbed and used by your body?

On a daily basis, our bodies create new muscle, skin and bone.

The body uses nerve signals and chemical messages to tell the body how to keep itself sustained and alive. How can we expect our bodies to do all this without fuel?

Fuel for the body must include at least 30 vitamins and minerals your body cannot produce on its own and therefore must access from nutrients. Vitamins and minerals are essential nutrients because of the hundreds of roles they play within your body. They heal wounds, keep bones strong, make you less susceptible to getting sick, repair cellular damage and convert your food into energy. You need vitamins to keep your body alive and well.

While vitamin supplements can be beneficial and are often necessary, the best way to obtain the vitamins and minerals your body needs is through food sources. This is because your body is best able to absorb the minerals and vitamins you need through what you eat. This is especially true for people who don't get all they need from food sources because of dietary restrictions such as lactose intolerance, vegetarians, vegans, etc.

Some great foods which are high in essential nutrients are proteins, whole grains, leafy greens and fruits. Let's take a look at which of these foods are the best for your body in terms of vitamin content, and why.

Vitamin A (and beta-carotene) is essential for all individuals, but is especially important in growing children. It creates healthy teeth and bones, promotes growth, helps the body resist infection and improves the body's cell structure and eyesight. The best sources of this vitamin come from dairy products, fish liver oils, carrots and dark-green leafy vegetables such as kale and spinach.

Vitamin B-1 (thiamine) is what helps the body digest and effectively use carbohydrates as fuel within the body. This vitamin also aids in keeping your nervous system functioning normally. Ways in which you can obtain this vitamin are through whole grains, brown rice, beans, peas, seeds and nuts, organ meats and lean pork.

Vitamin B-2 (riboflavin) prevents sores and swelling in your mouth and tongue. It also contributes to your body's functioning by helping to form enzymes to allow the process of oxidation to occur in your cells. Ways to get this vitamin include dairy products, meats, poultry, fish and green vegetables, particularly broccoli, turnip greens, asparagus and spinach.

Vitamin B-3 (niacin) is responsible for the health of your skin, your nervous and digestive systems, production of sex hormones and the detoxification of pollutants and alcohol in the body. You can get this vitamin by eating lean meats, fish, poultry and whole grains.

Vitamin B-6 (pyridoxine) is the vitamin responsible for the production of hemoglobin in your blood. You can obtain this vitamin by eating meats and whole grains.

Vitamin B-12 aids many areas of the body. It is responsible for the healthy functioning of your nervous system, the development of red blood cells, the production of genetic material in cells, and your body's efficient use of carbohydrates and folic acid from foods. Fish, dairy products, organ meats, beef, pork and eggs provide this vitamin.

Biotin is needed for the body to break down fatty acids in carbohydrates and helps the body get rid of wastes that occur from breakdown of proteins. This vitamin can be found in nuts, whole grains, vegetables, fruits, dairy products and organ meats.

Folic acid is responsible for the vital metabolic processes in the body, as well as the growth and production of red blood cells in the body. This vitamin comes from green leafy vegetables, oranges, beans, peas, rice, eggs and liver.

Pantothenic acid aids in the body's use of fats, carbohydrates and vitamins and contributes to the body's nervous system functions. This vitamin exists in organ meats, eggs and whole grains.

Vitamin D is most important for strong bones because of its ability to help the body absorb calcium and phosphorus from the digestive tract.

Vitamin D3 (Cholecalciferol) the most complete form of Vitamin D is made when the skin is exposed to the sun. Sunshine is a significant source; just 20 minutes per day is all you need. In addition, sunshine prevents depression (another added bonus.)

Include foods in your diet that contain vitamin D like fish--think Wild Salmon, cod liver oil, eggs, fresh fruits and vegetables.

Vitamin D is absolutely necessary for good health and research shows the list of benefits just keeps on growing.

Vitamin E is necessary for normal brain function, formation of red blood cells, and protection against pollutants in the body. This vitamin can be found in whole grains, green leafy vegetables and eggs.

Vitamin K is essential for aiding your blood in clotting. Vitamin K comes from green leafy vegetables and dairy products.

Enjoy your essential nutrients by eating a healthy and well-balanced diet with a variety of fruits and veggies.

WONDERS of WATER

Approximately 60-75% of your body weight is water. It is needed to flush out toxins and bring nutrients to your cells.

Dehydration occurs when your body does not get enough water to carry out routine functions.

Even mild dehydration can drain your energy and make you tired.
Rule of thumb: drink at least (8)-8 ounce glasses of water daily.
Consume more if you have exercised heavily, or been out in the sun for a period of time.
In addition, drink at least one glass of water for each alcoholic beverage that you consume.

Quality Counts

There are many different types of water available to us, so it can be confusing to choose the type with the most health benefits and is the least troubling for our bodies. The three issues to avoid are waters that have been stripped of minerals, water that has chlorine and chemicals and water that has BPA toxins.

Tap water, the water that comes out of faucets already treated, is not ideal for drinking because it has been processed and does not include the minerals your body needs. It also has been purified with chlorine and often has added fluoride, which studies suggest can lead to cancer.

Note: Unfiltered water may contain heavy metals, low levels of pharmaceuticals, and possibly dangerous pathogens.

Distilled water, water that has been vaporized and then collected, is also not ideal, because of the lack of minerals left behind during the distilling process.

Carbon filtering uses activated carbon to remove contaminants and impurities. It's an inexpensive and relatively easy way to filter out many contaminates found in ordinary tap water. It reduces chlorine and helps water taste better but does not remove minerals that may be associated with hard water.

Reverse osmosis water has been forced through a filter that removes particles and pollutants. The health advantage R.O. water has over tap water is that the R.O. system does remove some unhealthy contaminants. It is the only type of filter that will remove calcium and magnesium, the minerals that cause hard water. (Check to see if this may be a problematic issue where you live.)
With this type of water, you will not be drinking the needed minerals because they have been removed through filtering. Also, this process can get pricy and may require a plumber for installation. This water also tends to be acidic.
Bottled waters are not great for a number of reasons. First, disposable plastic containers contain BPA toxins that can cause diseases in our bodies. In addition, many bottled waters are often

just purified tap water that have chemicals and lack the minerals our bodies need.

Bottled water also has detrimental effects on the environment, because bottling and shipping water requires so many resources compared to drinking water from the source. If you must drink bottled water, use reusable glass, or metal containers rather than disposable plastic ones.

The best water out of all of these options to drink, is naturally clean water full of naturally occurring minerals. This can come from sources such as well water, natural spring water, artesian water and mineral water.

<u>**Some excellent ways to flavor water**</u>
Add mint leaves
Squeeze in some lemon, lime or citrus fruit
Add some cooling cucumber or
frozen strawberries, mango, blueberries etc.

Use your imagination.

Remember to Ditch the Diet Soda—nothing good there for you just a bunch of exotoxins-aka-crap.
YUCK

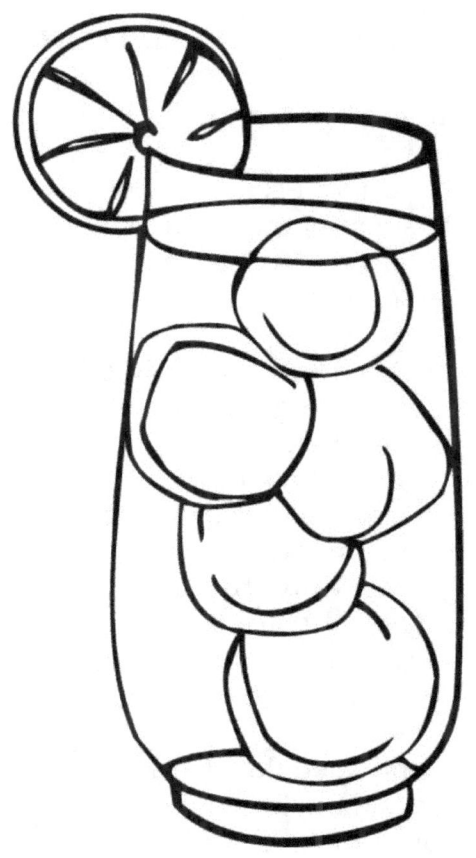

*"Pure water is the world's first
and foremost medicine."
~Slovakian Proverb*

SLEEP LIKE A BABY

If you want to find a way to lose weight faster, and you think there is nothing new under the sun, then what I'm about to tell you will really make you nod off.
Getting enough sleep each night is so important when you consider your body uses this time to repair itself and round out your path to better health.

According to Dr. Kenneth Goodrick at Baylor University, a good night's sleep is also a vital ingredient for weight loss.
This is not the only fascinating connection between sleep and weight gain. Researchers have found there are two hormones involved. Leptin, a hormone that suppresses appetite, and ghrelin, which increases food intake and is thought to play a role in long-term regulation of body weight. Sleep deprivation lowers the levels of leptin and raises levels of ghrelin.

In addition, some people drink several caffeinated beverages a day, which has an adverse effect on sleep quality. It's a double whammy!

What is a good night's sleep? Participants in a U.S. study who got less than 4 hours of sleep each night were 73 percent more likely to be obese than those who sleep between 7 and 9 hours a night, the recommended amount. Those who slept only 5 hours each night were 50 percent more likely to be overweight, and those who slept 6 hours a night were 23 percent more likely to be overweight.

In reality, sleep deprivation is taking a serious toll on our overall health.

A sleep deficit of merely 3 or 4 hours in a week may have a direct bearing on the following:

Obesity
Heart disease
Hypertension
Diabetes
Immune function
Cognitive performance
Longevity

Some Easy-Peasy tips for a good night's sleep:

Check your troubles at the door. They will be there for you tomorrow anyway, and you can deal with them better after a good night's sleep.

Create a peaceful atmosphere. Use some lavender oil, take a warm bath or sip a calming herbal tea. Listen to some tranquil sounds. Try some deep breathing exercises or nighttime meditation.

Cut the caffeine by noon. Better yet, cut it out altogether.

Avoid eating for at least 3 hours before bedtime.

Too much alcohol often results in a less restful sleep.

Get Un-Plugged ... Turn off the television and laptop at least an hour before bedtime.

Did you know?

Sex decreases the production of cortisol (which induces stress), and can put your body in a more relaxed state.

It's official, for good health we all need to wake up and get a good night sleep!

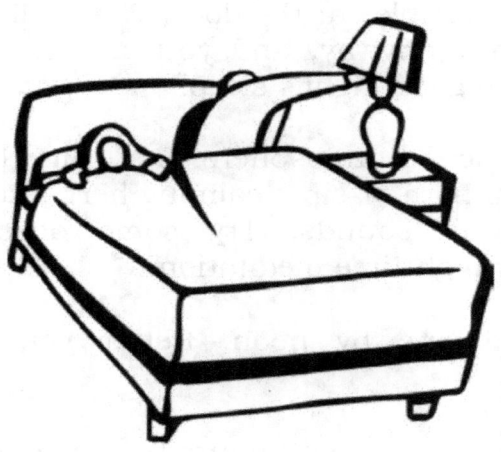

CHAPTER 3

DANGER AHEAD: PARTY PITFALLS

While I will always say, the best way to eat is with family and friends where you can enjoy, relax and feel at home, there are often occasions where partying with panache is the necessary standard of dining etiquette. Whether hosting a dining event of your own design or suffering through the ever-popular networking or job interview dinner, maintaining a particular style of class can make a difference in how people perceive you throughout the event.

Studies show that over 50% of the way in which others perceive you is determined by the message your body language sends, rather than what you communicate verbally. Therefore, it is essential you are regularly sending the right message through your actions throughout the night in order to make the best impression possible. A lot of pressure right? Well, not if you break the issue at hand down to some simple, easy to remember steps.

First, remember your mission. You are not at this event to gorge on free food; you are not there to get sloppy or drunk. The reason you are at the event is to entertain those around you, either for the purpose of hosting or networking. Focus on the impression you are making on those around you, not the nature of your stomach or an objective to overindulge. If eating a bit before hand to take the edge off an empty stomach and keep yourself from getting tipsy from a social drink is necessary so you can concentrate on your goals for the evening, go for it.

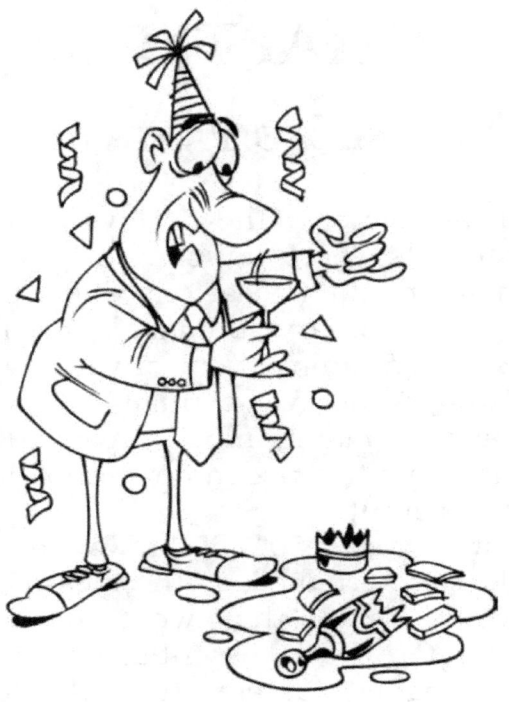

The second most important rule is to not get sloppy. First and foremost, don't get sloppy drunk-OMG! Let's focus on staying in control. Remind yourself that you have a two drink maximum for the evening or one drink if you're more of a lightweight; the purpose of the evening is not to get blasted. Don't get sloppy with your eating. Avoid foods that you know will give you trouble and make a mess, think saucy, and don't heap up your plate with tons of food. You can always go back for seconds, while still being presentable and able to be engaged with the people around you.

Third, make yourself available to the people around you. Don't hang out around the food table or bar. Engage with everyone in the room. Make your body language open and inviting. To do this your right hand should always be free to shake the hands of other people, so you must learn to balance your drink and food in your left hand. Make sure you finish each conversation conclusively before you go on to speaking with a new person, so no one feels dismissed. This might sound like a lot to remember, but to make a great impression at your next event, it is absolutely necessary.

WINE DOWN

So this is a bit of GOOD NEWS!

Arthur Agatston, MD, cardiologist and creator of the popular South Beach diet, encourages patients who enjoy alcohol also to drink it with meals.

"Alcohol can stimulate the appetite, so it is better to drink it with food. When alcohol is mixed with food, it can slow the stomach's emptying time and potentially decrease the amount of food consumed at a meal," asserts Dr. Agatston. His drink of choice is red wine due to the antioxidant resveratrol. However, he agrees that any alcohol in limited quantity will provide the same health benefit.

A few studies have found that people who drink alcohol in moderation have lower rates of heart disease, and might even live longer than those who abstain.

It is believed that the primary benefit of alcohol comes from its ability to raise HDL cholesterol levels, the "good" type that helps sweep cholesterol deposits out of your arteries and protects against a heart attack.

In particular, red wine might offer the greatest benefit for lowering heart disease risk and death because it contains - resveratrol - that has antioxidant properties and might protect artery walls.

On the flip-side drinking too much alcohol can actually increase your risk for heart disease and stroke, raise blood pressure, contribute to obesity, and increase the levels of fats called triglycerides in the blood.

The health benefits associated with drinking in moderation are also similar for beer, wine and spirits. The primary factor associated with health and longevity appears to be the alcohol itself.

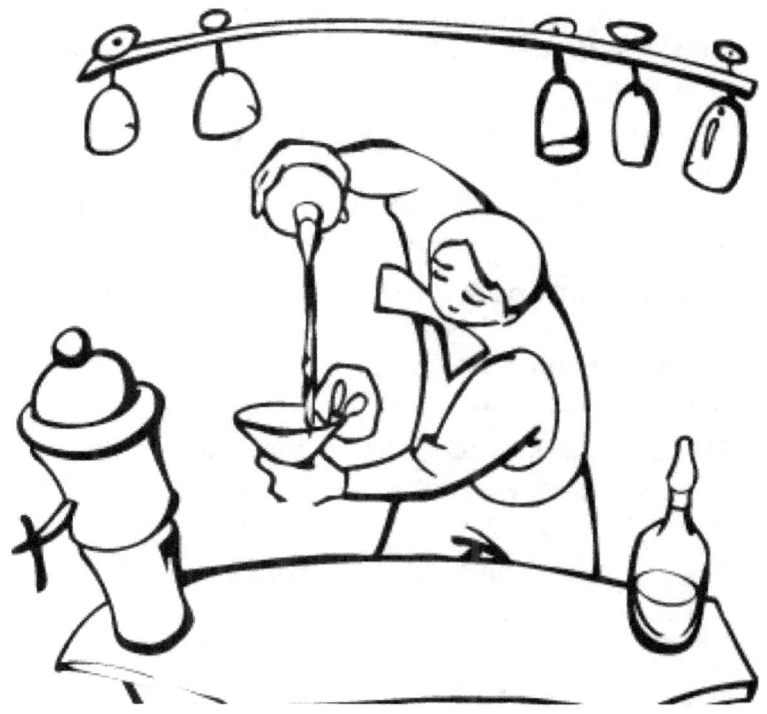

Some Tips for Drinking in Moderation

- Know your limit. It's best to stop at 1 or 2.
- Eat food while you drink. Food, especially high protein food such as meat, preferably organic, unprocessed cheese, and almonds, will help slow the absorption of alcohol into your body.

- Sip your drink. Don't Gulp! When you gulp a drink, you lose the pleasure of savoring its flavors and aromas, and you end up looking like an idiot.

- Don't participate in "chugging" contests or other drinking games.

  (I don't need to tell you these things—if I do, you may have other problems beyond the scope of this book.)

- Accept a drink only when you really want one. Don't be afraid to ask for a non-alcohol beverage instead. If that doesn't work, "lose" your drink by setting it down somewhere and leaving it.

- Skip a drink now and then. Having a non-alcoholic drink between alcoholic ones will help keep your blood alcohol content level down, as does spacing out your alcoholic drinks.

- Drink at least one glass of water for each serving of alcohol, in addition to the recommended daily water intake. Alcohol is dehydrating.

- Keep active; don't just sit around and drink. If you stay active, you tend to drink less and may be more aware of any effects alcohol may be having on you.

- Beware of unfamiliar drinks. Some drinks, such as zombies and other fruit drinks, can be deceiving as the alcohol content is not detectable. Therefore, it is difficult to space them properly.

- Use alcohol carefully in connection with pharmaceuticals. Ask your physician or pharmacist about any precautions or prohibitions and follow any advice received.

Remember...
A glass of white or red wine, a bottle of beer, and a shot of whiskey or other distilled spirits all contain equivalent amounts of alcohol. A standard drink is:

- A 12-ounce bottle or can of regular beer

- A 5-ounce glass of wine

- A 1&1/2 ounce shot of 80 proof distilled spirits (either straight or in a mixed drink)

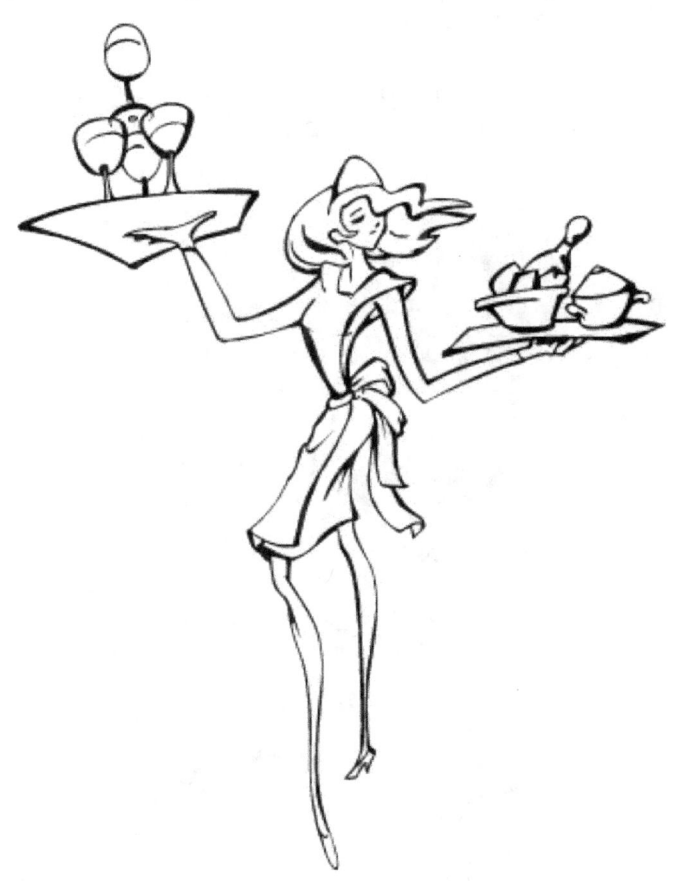

CHAPTER 4

Quit Yer Bitchin in the Kitchen

Kitchen Clean-Up Time:
Refrigerator Re-Do and Pantry Purge

If you want to eat better, get healthier, shed the excess weight it's time to purge the junk.

Take a picture of your refrigerator right now.
No fussing or primping, just DO IT!

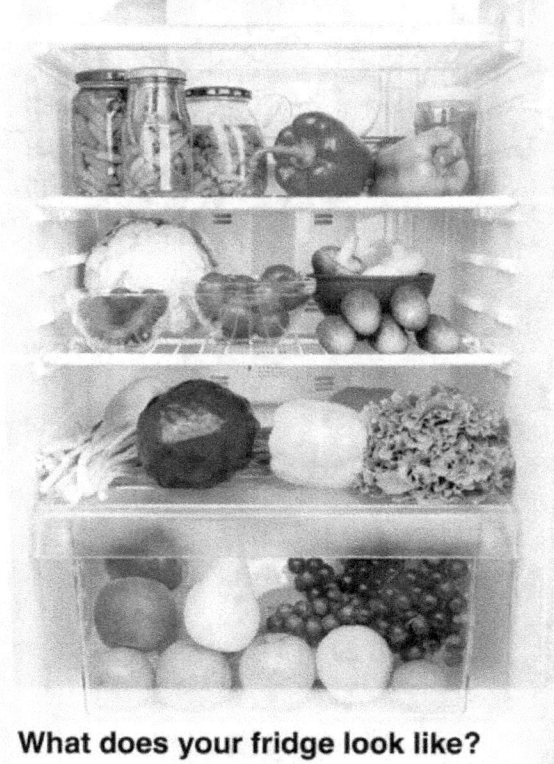

What does your fridge look like?

What do you see?

Is it organized and clean?
Or...do you have to scrape "gunk" off of the sides?

What the hell is it?

Either unidentifiable by its appearance or you
don't understand the label ...
time to toss it.

You can *live* without it!

What does your pantry look like?

Are you happy with what you see?

Pick up a box, can, etc. from your pantry or
refrigerator. Chances are that there are several
ingredients that you cannot pronounce or have never
heard of. When was the last time you made a home
cooked meal which called for hydrogenated palm
kernel oil? How about butylated hydroxytoluene
(BHT)?
Both of these examples are known to cause toxicity of
vital organs in humans and are hiding in many of the
processed foods on grocery store shelves. Do your
research. There are thousands of known carcinogens
lurking in processed foods, which can cause
everything from tumors to mental disorders, from
severe migraines to skin rashes. I think a good amount
of you would be surprised by how seemingly unrelated
symptoms clear up once you clean up your diet.

It's time to do a Pantry Purge

Do you swear you're going to get around to clean it out, but then come up with every excuse not to?

No more excuses, let's get started:

> Dump everything with high fructose corn syrup,
> artificial color or flavoring and
> words that make no sense.

> Say buh-bye
> to those sugar laden cereals!

> Remember to check for expiration dates.

> Why did you buy this crap
> in the first place?

> Out of sight, out of mind.
> Ditch the junk food.

It is best to keep those temptation foods out of the home and enjoy the occasional indulgence when you're dining out with friends.

Raw almonds, walnuts, pumpkin seeds are some terrific options that will stay fresh for a few months and are a wonderful substitute from those unhealthy snacks. Add in a bit of dried fruit, and you have your own homemade trail mix.

Once you've purged your pantry, categorize your remaining items in a manner similar to a store.

For example:

EVOO and Coconut oils
Spices
Nuts & Seeds

Baking Items such as Almond flour, Shredded coconut, Unsweetened 100% cacao (powdered and organic), etc.

Reduce the use of canned foods since most cans are lined with BPA-containing resin. However, due to the convenience, there are a few acceptable choices such as:
organic tomato sauce, coconut milk, pumpkin puree. I prefer to see items that are "healthier choices" in glass containers. Check the label, eventually; you will get the hang of it.

Create an area where the kiddos can reach for healthy food choices.

Tip: Physically remove tempting food items from your home and office.

Reasons to Shun SUGAR

When you think of sugar, you think of happy things. It's things you put on birthday cakes, treats and things for special occasions.

Think again!

The average American consumes about two and a half pounds of sugar per week, which is equal to about 5 cups.

It is found lurking in so many of our manufactured foods, and it messes with your metabolism.

Think about all of the places sugar is hiding. For example: an iced latte contains about 7 teaspoons of sugar, a single serving of yogurt can have as much as 30 grams equivalent to 7 ½ teaspoons and it also is in "so-called" healthy products such as cereals, raisin bran and breads.

Government guidelines recommend no more than 25 grams or 6 ¼ teaspoons of added sugars per day.

Sugar may be injuring our liver and metabolism, weakening our immune system and putting us at risk of multiple lifestyle related diseases and conditions.

When we have excess sugar in our bodies, it is stored in our liver as FAT. Everyone knows too much sugar causes weight gain. It can lead to things like insulin resistance, metabolic syndrome and diabetes.

Labels can be very confusing; sugar isn't always listed as sugar. There are many common names for sugar that include:

Granulated sugar
Brown sugar
Confectioners' sugar
Corn sugar
Raw sugar

Beware of words that end in OSE and OL such as:
Dextrose
Galactose
Maltose
Saccharose
Xylose

Mannitol
Xylitol

Unfortunately, there are many more words that mean sugar. This will also include: corn syrup, cane juice, fruit juice concentrate, honey, syrup, molasses and more.

What about high fructose corn syrup (HFCS)?
According to the United States Department of Agriculture,
Americans consume approximately 35 pounds of high fructose corn syrup annually.
Many years ago concerns were raised in regard to high fructose corn syrup and the nations growing obesity problem.
Manufacturers love it - it is cheap (you are not) and it extends shelf life.
Read your labels carefully, high fructose corn syrup shows up everywhere, even canned soups and the most unsuspecting places.

If you must have sugar, avoid refined or manufactured sugar and look for the most natural sources such as: organic or raw sugar, USDA honey, molasses or organic stevia are regarded as safer alternatives in small amounts.

*So what's the skinny on artificial sweeteners
as an alternative to sugar?*

I strongly advise against anything artificial,
especially fake sugar products such as aspartame
and sucralose.
It tricks the pleasure center of your brain and as
you are still digesting you end up feeling hungrier
and experience more cravings. The "fake sugar"
can actually ***promote weight gain.***
The opposite of what you want.
In addition, artificial sugar can aggravate your
intestinal lining: resulting in digestive problems,
which include diarrhea, worsens Crohn's disease
and can cause an upset stomach.

What about fruit?
Sugars in fruit are naturally occurring and contain
vitamins and essential fiber.

Don't go crazy with too much fruit though as it
can sabotage weight loss goals.

PASS on the SALT

Studies show cutting down on sodium in your diet can lower blood pressure and reduce your risk of stroke, heart failure and other health problems.

The U.S. Food and Drug Administration recommend most people consume less than 2,300 mg. of sodium each day. That's only one teaspoon. People with certain medical conditions and the elderly should limit their intake to 1,500 mg.

However, the average American consumes about 3,400 mg of sodium per day. Way more than the recommended daily limits.

Isn't sea salt healthier than table salt?

Sea salt is generally marketed as a "natural" and "healthier" alternative.

The main differences between sea salt and table salt are in taste, texture and processing. Sea salt has a stronger flavor. However, what people should remember is that both sea salt and table salt have the same amount of sodium by weight.

Should I just stop using the salt shaker?

It does help to avoid adding salt to your food at the table, but, unfortunately, a major part of the sodium in American diets (approximately 80 percent) comes from processed and packaged foods. These foods can be high in sodium even if they don't taste salty.

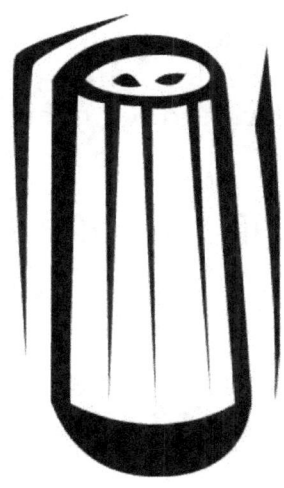

Processed foods include:
- Frozen meals
- Canned or pickled foods
- Snack food
- Deli meat
- Cheese
- Condiments, sauces and dressings
- Breads
- Cereals

By now you should understand processed foods have no place in our weight loss goals or have any health benefits. Stay away.

By the way, "table salt" or sodium chloride is a chlorinated, processed salt that is stripped of all of its minerals.

Substitute a high-quality salt such as pink Himalayan sea salt, which is not chlorinated or processed, and none of the minerals have been stripped away.

If you are on a sodium-restricted diet, consider the use of Sea Kelp, which has lower sodium content.

Remember: too much salt makes you retain water, so you will look and feel BLOATED.

Microwaves: Magic or Madness?

Just about every home has one. How safe is this once touted modern day marvel. Granted, they are great time savers. The question here is, how safe are these machines for humans?

Cooking food in the microwaves is one of the major causes of ill health and the harmful effects of it are ignored mostly. The harmful change that microwave ovens bring to the molecules of food is creating new forms of life that are called "radiolytic compounds." These compounds are a mutation that is so far unknown in the natural world.

The microwave that you often use is not just a heating tool. It is way much cancerous and toxic. For the long term and regular usage, microwaves can lead to some serious health issues. Instead of saving some of your time, try the simple cooking methods and stay happier and healthier.

One of the dangers that people face because of microwaves is their leakage problem. This issue is so serious that FDA has set some strict limitations for the manufacturers. But no matter what, the seals of a microwave tend to break once it gets old and leakage starts. This is actually very bad because the energy inside a microwave is too much. Studies showed that a frequency of over 10 hertz can harm your body while a microwave contains the frequency of 2.45 BILLION hertz.

Possible Diseases Caused By Microwave:

The first scientist to study the dangers of microwaves was Hans Hertel. He studied how cooking in a microwave depletes and degrades the nutrients of food. He found out that eating the food cooked in a microwave can cause a decrease in the count of white blood cells, and a decrease in hemoglobin. Further, eating microwaved food can lead to several heart diseases, anemia, degenerative issues and even cancer.

Russia was a country that didn't appreciate this harmful machine. In fact, they banned it in 1976 after doing their research about the biological effects of microwave ovens. They ran experiments on the food treated in microwave ovens and discovered a link between stomach related cancer and the microwave.

Exposure to BPA:

In addition to this, when you use plastic wraps and plastic containers to heat your food, you get all the harmful chemicals in your food like BPA and xenoestrogens which are considered cancer causing agents.

Studies showed that BPA, which is used in manufacturing of polycarbonate and other types of plastics, could cause erectile dysfunction and reproductive issues. This has also been linked with the cardiovascular problems and even diabetes.

You might be thinking that you just use your microwave oven to heat the leftovers, and it is not harmful. This is a totally wrong concept. The food you heat in the microwave is not heated evenly and is a mixture of cool as well as the super-heated spots. Those cold spots can harbor bacteria, and you might end up with the food poisoning.

Therefore, it is recommended for you to stop cooking food in the microwaves and if you have no other option, then try not using it regularly.

TRUTH: I gave up using a microwave eight years ago. I don't miss it.

CHAPTER 5

Savvy Supermarket Shopping

Many of you have heard about shopping the perimeter of the grocery store. This means exactly what it says; most grocery stores are designed so the fresh produce, fresh meats, fish, dairy, etc. are on the perimeter of the store. The rest of the store, think snacks, processed foods, packaged items, canned goods, candies, breads, and sodas are located in the inside aisles. This is the part of the store you want to avoid as much as possible. As a general rule, you are almost always better off sticking to the perimeter, where you will find the most wholesome food and filling your grocery carts with fresh foods.

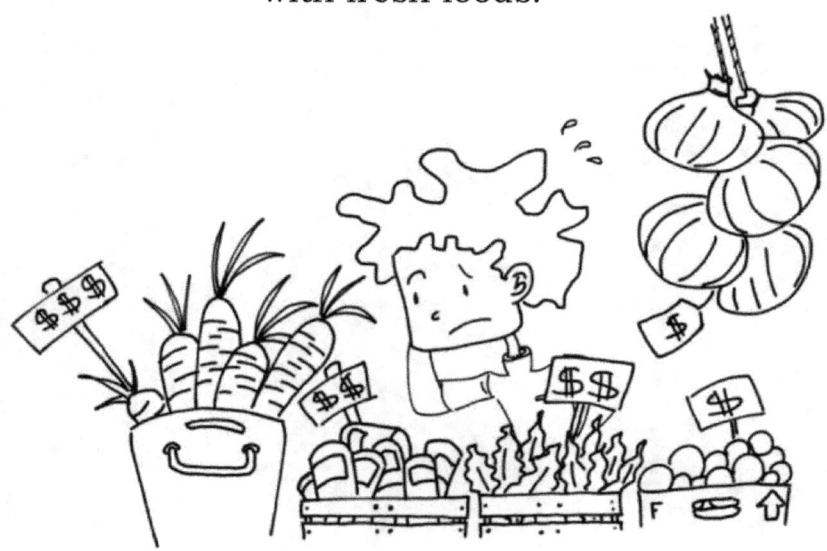

Tip #1   *NEVER* go food shopping when you are hungry and always make a list of food items prior to shopping.

Tip #2   Your shopping goal is only to purchase items that you can consume within a week or less. Bring home only what you feel good about eating.

Tip #3   Don't succumb to the hype or fancy marketing.

Become a LABEL DETECTIVE

If you can't read or pronounce it … Put it Down
Watch out for Artificial Flavoring or Coloring
or "Artificial" Anything
Be on the Lookout for Hidden Sugars
Look for Low-Sodium Alternatives (federal guidelines cap sodium intake to 1500mg/day)

Avoid lifeless, depleted, highly processed, nutrient deficient food.

According to the Environmental Working Group (EWG), a nonprofit organization that advocates policies that protect global and individual health, not all produce needs to be purchased organic.

The "**Clean 15**" list had the lowest pesticide load, and consequently are the safest conventionally grown crops to consume from the standpoint of pesticide contamination. These include:

- Avocados
- Sweet corn
- Pineapples
- Cabbage
- Sweet peas (frozen)
- Onions
- Asparagus
- Mangoes
- Papayas
- Kiwi
- Eggplant
- Grapefruit
- Cantaloupe (domestic)
- Cauliflower
- Sweet potatoes

"**Dirty Dozen Plus**" list include the highest pesticide load, making them the most important to buy or grow organic versions:

- Apples
- Blueberries (domestic)
- Strawberries
- Grapes
- Celery
- Peaches
- Spinach
- Sweet bell peppers
- Nectarines (imported)
- Cucumbers
- Cherry tomatoes
- Snap peas (imported)

- Potatoes
- Hot peppers

To learn more, I highly suggest taking a look at their website: http://www.ewg.org

Purchasing Produce – (PLU codes)

Did you ever notice those little round stickers on your produce? They are called the Product LookUp or PLU for short.
The code on the sticker will tell you whether the produce is Organically Grown, Conventionally Grown or Genetically Modified.

Now look at the digits on the code—if it is:

<u>4 digits starts with #3 or #4</u> it is
CONVENTIONALLY GROWN
(refer to the dirty dozen clean 15 chart – if the item is on the clean 15, and budget is an issue, it is safe to purchase conventionally. If it is on the Dirty Dozen—stick with Organic.)

<u>5 digits starts with #9</u> it is
ORGANICALLY GROWN
Best Choice-the produce has been grown using no synthetic fertilizers or pesticides.

<u>5 digits starts with #8</u> it is a
GENETICALLY MODIFIED ORGANISM
(also known as GMO)
Don't buy it. Put it down and run for the hills, it is **J-U-N-K**.

A bit about Organics

100 percent organic - Product must be either completely organic or made of all organic ingredients.

Organic - Product must be at least 95 percent organic to use this term.

"made with organic ingredients" – Product must contain at least 70 percent organic ingredients.

In order for a product to use the USDA Organic Seal, it must be Organic or 100% Organic.

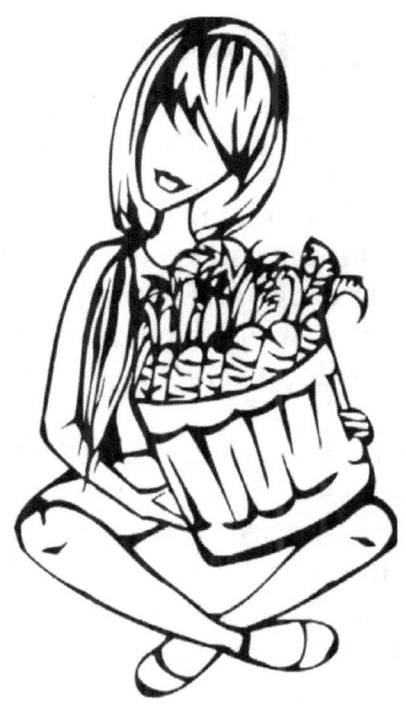

**Tip: Choose fresh, wholesome foods grown
locally and seasonally.**

GMO-No Go!

I want to give you the opportunity to decide for yourself if GMOs are something you want to include on YOUR plate. In more than 60 countries around the world, including Australia, Japan, and all of the countries in the European Union, there are significant restrictions or outright bans on the production and sale of GMOs.

So what's all this hype about GMOs, which are everywhere in food these days, are they horrible for your health? Are the rumors true? What is a GMO? The full name of "GMO" is "genetically modified organism" (sometimes referred to as "genetically engineered organisms"). This is an organism whose genetic material has been altered using genetic engineering techniques. Genetically modified foods are meat products and plants which have had their DNA artificially altered in a laboratory by genes from other plants, animals, viruses, or bacteria.

GMOs are not created to alleviate famine or alter foods in a positive way for consumers, but rather make production of food easier and more viable for the companies that sell it. Some studies estimate that over 75% of all processed foods sold in the U.S. contain GMO ingredients, particularly corn, soy, canola, cottonseed, sugar, beef and dairy products. Companies are sneaky in the ways in which they get around leaving customers in the dark about these ingredients and the United

States government does not require labeling of these ingredients on products, so consumption of GMOs goes largely unnoticed.

So what's so bad about eating these products? Not to mention the harmful effects they have on farmers and the environment, GMOs are suspected to have terrible effects on the health of consumers. In fact, studies of animals that have eaten GMOs have experienced reproductive problems, poor immunity, accelerated aging, blood sugar imbalances and harmful effects on major organs.

One reason GMOs are so unhealthy is the amount and type of harmful pesticides that have been sprayed on these food products. Because GMO plants are bred to be resistant to pesticides, companies can use pesticides with higher toxins in greater amounts without consequence. Some issues in humans that have arisen since the introduction of GMOs, although no studies exist to prove that GMOs are truly the cause of these issues, include allergies, infertility, birth defects, digestive issues, imbalances in gut bacteria, cancers and tumors.

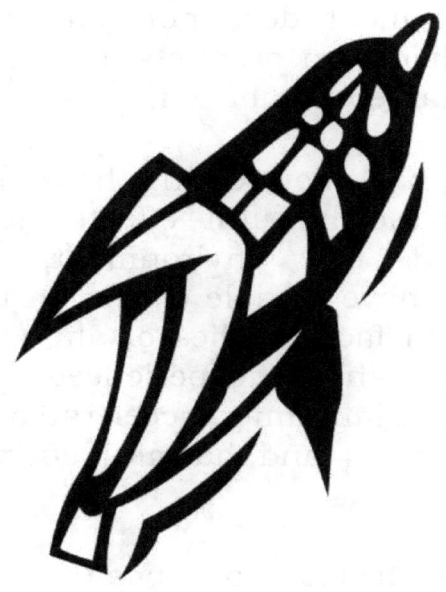

So how can GMOs be avoided? Buy organic, because these products do not include any GMO ingredients. Look for non-GMO product seals on the foods you choose. Avoid products with ingredients which are often high in GMOs such as dairy products, sugars, corn, soy, canola, cottonseed, sugar beets, Hawaiian papaya, zucchini and yellow squash. Look for shopping guides that specifically tell you what you can buy that's GMO-free on many GMO-free websites. Some of my faves are below:

http://www.nongmoproject.org

http://www.nongmoshoppingguide.com

EAT THE RAINBOW

Know you color Wheel

When it comes to healthy weight loss, make sure your plate is piled high with a range of colorful fruit and vegetables. You will naturally create more balance and health-filled menus.

Why? Color not only brightens your mood but also your diet. Load your plate with fruit and veggies like a box of crayons in colors such as red, yellow, orange, blue, purple, white and green. You will also be filling up on power packed phytonutrients. Phytonutrients are naturally occurring chemicals which combat disease.

In "What Color Is Your Diet?" by David Heber, MD, Ph.D., and Susan Bowerman R.D. attempted to group foods according to their predominant phytochemical group, coding plant foods into color categories.

Blue/Purple
The blue/purple hues in foods are due primarily to their anthocyanin content. Anthocyanins are antioxidants that are found naturally in a number of foods. Anthocyanins are the pigments that give their rich coloring. Some examples: berries, red onions, eggplant, plums, kidney beans, pomegranates.
They are believed to be heart healthy.

Did you know: blueberries are considered to have the highest antioxidant activity of all foods?

Green
Chlorophyll colors green fruits and vegetables Cruciferous veggies such as broccoli and cabbage contain the phytochemicals, which may have anticancer properties and are excellent sources of vitamin K, folic acid and potassium.
Vitamin K is essential in blood clot formation. Diets high in potassium are associated with lowering blood pressure, and there is an inverse relationship between cruciferous vegetables and cancer, especially colon and bladder cancers.
Examples: Broccoli, cabbage, bok choy, Brussels sprouts.

Yellow/Green
A variation of the green color category, these foods exhibit a richness in lutein, says Bowerman. "Lutein is particularly beneficial for eye health," she says.
Another plus in grabbing some yellow/green fruits and veggies at the grocery store is it's a rich source of vitamin C.
Examples: Avocado, kiwifruit, spinach and other leafy greens, pistachios, peas.

Red
Lycopene is the predominant pigment in reddish fruits and veggies, according to Bowerman. A carotenoid, lycopene is a powerful antioxidant that has been associated with a reduced risk of some cancers, especially prostate cancer, and protection

against heart attacks. Look for tomato-based products for the most concentrated source of this phytochemical.

According to information from Produce for Better Health Foundation, cooked tomato sauces are associated with greater health benefits than the uncooked version because the heating process allows all carotenoids, including lycopene, to be more easily absorbed by the body,
In addition to vitamin C and folate, red fruits and vegetables are also sources of flavonoids, which reduce inflammation and have antioxidant properties.
Examples: Tomatoes and tomato products, watermelon, pink grapefruit, guava, and cranberries.

Yellow/Orange
Orange group foods are also rich in beta-carotene, which are particularly good antioxidants and a good source of vitamin C.
These foods are commonly considered the eyesight foods because they contain vitamin A in which eyesight is dependent upon.
Examples: Carrots, mangos, cantaloupe, winter squash, sweet potatoes, pumpkins, and apricots.

No Color? No Problem
While color can give clients a general idea about what lies beneath eggplant's exterior, a food's hue does not tell all, and it is certainly not an exclusive indicator of phytochemical content. While some phytochemicals are pigments that give color,

others are colorless.

"The largest class of phytochemicals are the flavonoids, which for the most part are colorless," explains Bowerman. "Flavonoids are potent antioxidants, and these help the body to counteract free-radical formation. When free-radical damage goes unchecked, it can cause significant damage to body cells and tissues."

You'll get more enjoyment from eating when there's a variety of colors and flavors on your plate.

FABLE OF LABELS

Food labels are clever marketing tools designed to do one thing - SELL the product. There is so much confusion surrounding food labels I just want to clarify some of the mysteries behind it.

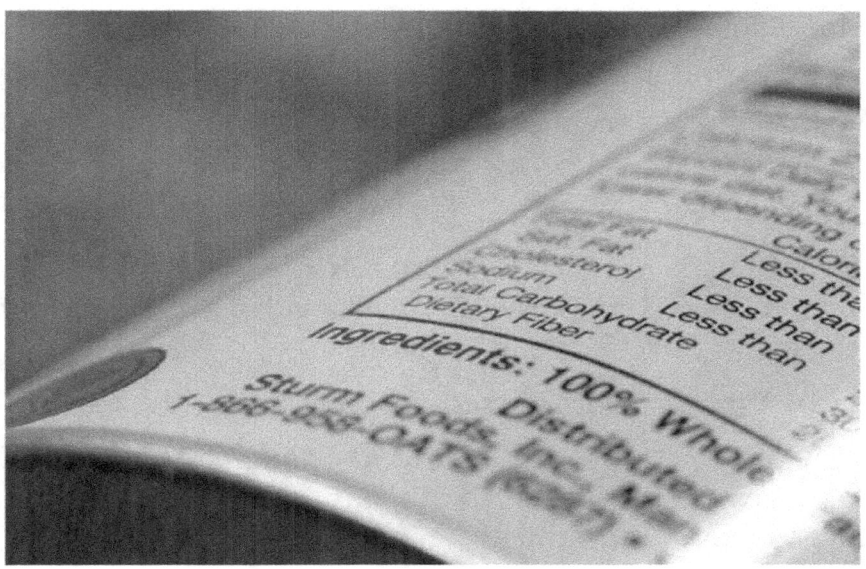

Some common "buzz" words to watch out for:

FAT-FREE - The product has less than .5 grams of fat per serving.

LOW FAT - The product has 3 grams or less of fat per serving.

REDUCED or LESS FAT - The product has at least 25% less fat per serving than the full-fat version.

Beware: Lower fat options often contain added sugars to make up for flavor loss.

71

LITE or LIGHT - This one is ambiguous and can have a number of meanings:

- the product has fewer calories or half the fat of the non-light version,

- the sodium content of a low-calorie, low-fat food is 50 percent less than the non-light version,

- a food is clearer in color (like light instead of dark corn syrup).

CALORIE FREE - The product has less than 5 calories per serving.

LOW CALORIE - The product has 40 calories or less per serving.

REDUCED or FEWER CALORIES - The product has at least 25 percent fewer calories per serving than the non-reduced version.

Other "trick" words used on labels include:

"Fortified," "enriched," "added," "extra", and "plus" usually mean the food has been altered or processed in some way.

"Fruit drinks" usually means little or no real fruit and a lot of sugar. Instead look for products that say "100% fruit juice."

"Made with wheat," or "rye," or "multi-grains" imply it's a good source of whole grains, but unfortunately, don't tell you how much whole grain is actually in the product. Look for the word "whole" before the grain to ensure you are actually getting a 100% whole-grain product.

"Natural" or "made from natural" simply means the manufacturer started with a natural source.

Once processed, the food may not resemble anything natural or pure.

"Organically grown," "organic," "pesticide-free," and "no artificial ingredients" say very little about the nutritional value or safety of the product. Trust only those labels that say "certified organically grown."

"Sugar-free," "sugarless," or "no added sugar" tells you nothing about sugar derivatives or sugar substitutes, which yield just as many calories as table sugar and may be more harmful to you than sugar.

Ingredient Lists

Okay, now that you know how to decode the front labels, the real proof is in the pudding, the ingredients list. Here's where you'll find the hidden saturated and trans fats, sugars, sodium, artificial flavorings, and refined grains. Ingredients are listed in order of most to least amounts. That means the first ingredient will be in the largest quantity. The second is the second most and so on.

When decoding the ingredients list label watch out for these "evildoer" ingredients whenever possible:

• Olestra: a fake fat that eliminates good vitamins from the system and can cause major digestive upset.

• "Enriched flour," "wheat flour," or "unbleached wheat flour," are all code words for refined flour with just a small amount of whole wheat added.

- "Partially hydrogenated" or "hydrogenated oils": code words for trans fats.

- Nitrates: used to preserve meats and have been linked to creating a powerful cancer-causing chemical in the body; found especially in luncheon meats.

- High fructose corn syrup: a fancy phrase for refined sugar. Other forms of sugar to watch out for in the ingredients list include: honey, molasses, fruit juice concentrate, evaporated cane juice, malt, dextrose, and, of course, sugar.

- Lard shortening: pure animal fat.

- Artificial food colorings: are chemicals used to add color to foods.

- Monosodium glutamate (MSG) : a form of sodium; other words which mean high sodium including brine, disodium phosphate, garlic salt, onion salt, sodium alginate, sodium benzoate, sodium caseinate, sodium hydroxide, sodium nitrate, sodium pectinate, sodium propionate, sodium sulfite, baking powder, baking soda, and soy sauce.

There are many more ingredients we could list, but in the interest of saving space, here's a rule of thumb: if a food item is packed with lots of ingredients that you can't pronounce, they are artificial sounding, and it includes trans fats, you should look for a better food choice. Try to stick with products that are made from whole foods, with little to no preservatives, and with little to no artificial sounding ingredients, and definitely no trans fats.

There are over 20,000 food items in the average grocery store, trying to find the truly healthy brands is like looking for a needle in a haystack, unless you know how to decode the labels on the packaged food items.

"Though no one can go back and make a brand new start, anyone can start from now and make a brand new ending." – Carl Bard

Gluten: Fact or Fiction?

Wary of wheat?

Wheat today is not the same wheat our grandparents baked with many years ago. Today's wheat has been hybridized to create dwarf wheat to increases output by tenfold on the same acre of land. This hybrid wheat protein has been dramatically altered, and it has not been tested for human safety.

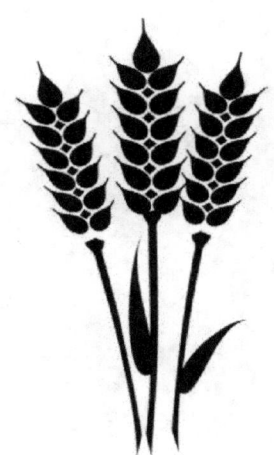

WHAT IS GLUTEN?

Gluten is what gives your favorite breads and bakery goods their chewy texture.

It is a protein found in wheat, barley, rye, spelt and sometimes oats. Gluten-free is another buzzword you have surely heard or seen at your local supermarket.

WHAT'S THE BIG DEAL?

I wondered the same thing. I grew up on a steady diet of white bread, pizza, pasta; you name it.

A small percentage of the population is affected by celiac disease, a severe autoimmune response triggered by the consumption of gluten. People with celiac disease must completely avoid gluten.

What I didn't know was gluten can cause a host of other health issues for the rest of us, such as eczema, asthma, abdominal cramps, bloating, skin issues, achy joints and more. By removing gluten from the diet, many people resolve a myriad of health issues and feel better.

WONDER IF WHEAT IS CAUSING ISSUES FOR YOU?

If you are curious, something easy you can do is remove wheat from your diet for a week and then reintroduce it. By taking this "wheat-free holiday," you will be able to see how your body reacts to gluten when you reintroduce it to your diet.

READ your labels. Just because a food is labeled "Gluten-Free" doesn't mean it is good for you. It still can be "junk food" that happens to be gluten-free.

CHAPTER 6

The Dish on Detoxification – What's the Big Deal?

WHAT ARE TOXINS?

Well, basically toxins can be grouped into three different sections. There are exogenous toxins, endogenous toxins and finally autogenous toxins.

Exogenous toxins are ones that are created from outside, or things that we eat. They can be residue from herbicides that are sprayed onto vegetables or fruit, but they can also be stimulants, alcohol, caffeine, too much sugar or fat in the body, the build up that has been caused by breathing in fumes that are in the air if you live in a city or big town.

Endogenous toxins are more complex. These often are formed in the bowel, and they are the residual waste that has been created after you have a virus or some kind of bacterial infection. So, you get an infection, you get 'better' and you think that life carries on as normal. Well, deep in the heart of your bowel, lots of little toxins are left over from the infection, and they just clog up the work that your bowel is trying to do. The only thing you can do to help your bowel is to get rid of them.

Finally, the last group of toxins is the autogenous toxins. These are all made by you. Everyone has these. They are simply a way of the body dumping out some refuse, as a result of the natural metabolic process. So they are completely natural, but they can still act as a barrier to your body working as well as it could.

WHY DETOX?

Detox removes toxins from your body. The goal of a detox diet or cleanse is to expel unnatural toxins from your body.

Fat cells store many toxins; losing excess fat releases these toxins so they can be eliminated.

We live in a very fast-paced world where many of us are now eating diets that are convenience oriented, processed and just plain lacking in nutrition.

Modern life bombards you with toxins, pollutants, chemicals, plastics, pesticides and other environmental contaminants. Sadly, all of this affects our water, food and air quality.

In addition, sugar, caffeine, alcohol and preservatives in our food, can wreak havoc on your body over time.

Billions of pounds of chemical pollutants are released into the environment over the course of a year. Sadly, it can enter our body through our skin, the air we breathe and the food we eat.

How can we possibly fuel our bodies' natural detoxification process? (Detoxification refers to our bodies' natural ability to remove toxins.)

Did you know that your body might be carrying around 5-10 pounds of toxicity-aka-inflammation? This can lead to headaches, weight gain, bloating, and disease.

Whether it is the toxic load of processed foods eaten, the drinks we indulge in, pollution, pesticides, personal care products and so on.

Now think about this over the course of a *LIFETIME*.

Combined toxins over time = A Big Mess

Just like our homes need a good seasonal cleaning, so does our body.

Cleansing is not just about what you eat, but also about the mental, emotional and spiritual properties that align with each season.
Just like ancient cultures have learned and taught for 1000's of years.

We can help our body by reducing the effects of toxicity that include:
• Avoid: additives, preservatives, unhealthy fats and processed junk

- If it's made in a plant, forget it.
  If it comes from a plant, go for it.
- Ditch the processed stuff
- Drink water...6-8 glasses every day
  Your body is up to 75% water, so quality and quantity count
- Eat fresh whole fruit and vegetables in their most natural state (preferably organic)
- Read labels – If you don't understand it, don't eat it
- Ease up on animal fats – Go organic or at least try the leanest cuts
- Eat safe fish ... preferably from cold water sources
- Eat-In more often, you can control what goes into your food and save money at the same time

Use an Air-Purifier
Change air conditioning filters often
Use a Hepa-Vac to reduce household allergens
Use personal care and household items that are non-toxic or organic

WHEN IS IT BEST TO DETOX?

You may read different things about the best time to detox, but in reality, there is only one best time to go through a detox program, and that is NOW. Some people like to detox at the beginning of each new season, because they think that it is a time for new beginnings, time to clean the home, yard and basically get fit for the coming season. But it is really ok to detox any time. After all, if you are thinking about detoxing in the fall and then you leave it till spring time, then you may well forget about it, so try to plan your detox for as soon as possible, to make sure that it actually happens.

There is only one time when detox may not be a good thing and that is if you are facing a really difficult time in your life, in terms of your health, or the health of a loved one, or if work or something in your life is particularly stressful. There is no point setting yourself up to fail, so try to build in a few days where you can just unwind, relax and have a nice easy time of it at the start of your detox. That way you are more likely to succeed and this makes the whole process just that bit more enjoyable and fun.

You also need to be aware that if you are living a toxic lifestyle at the moment, whereby you are eating lots of processed food, or sweet, fatty foods, drinking lots of alcohol or coffee or even just caffeine based drinks such as cola, then you will have to prepare your body for detox. That means you will have to cut down on caffeine, alcohol and other toxic foods, so that you do not feel withdrawal symptoms after you start your program. So if you are very toxic, start cutting down for a week before you actually initiate a detox program.

Poop - the Scoop

Not the most glamorous conversation here, but this topic really needs to be addressed.
Why? Because poop is a very state-of-the-art-way that says a lot about the state of our health. Time to pay attention.

So what's this stuff made of? For the most part water (approximately 75%) and the rest of it is a combination of dead and living bacteria, mucous and cells. Poop should have the consistency of peanut butter.

Is there an "ideal" poop? Just remember this - B.S. (Best Sh*t)
B is for brown, which is the ideal color, due to the bile secreted in our liver.
S is for shape, size, smell and sink. You should hear a "plop" when your poop hits the toilet, and it should sink. If the size is about 4-8 inches and resembles the shape of a snake and doesn't smell too much, give yourself a cheer. You have achieved the B.S. award. Do I hear any clapping out there? Well, it is a big feat.

How often is "normal?" This is widely debated, and I've seen many different answers to this question. This can range from person to person and culture to culture. How much or how often do you eat is also a consideration. A traditional approach suggests anything from 3 times per day to once every 3 days within the "normal" range. A holistic approach suggests at least once per day, preferably 2 or 3 times per day. If you think about the typical person eating 3 meals per day and doesn't eliminate for days, what happens?

It sits in your gut, where do all those toxins go? Ewwww - you choose here.

What to be on the lookout for? Floating poop, usually, indicates a high-fat content, a possible sign of malabsorption. Color may vary due to what foods you have consumed, but be clued into persistent changes, which can possibly spell trouble. If that is the case, see your healthcare professional.

The digestive process normally takes 24-72 hours from the time you eat and the journey through the esophagus, stomach, small and large intestine and finally out the exit.

Constipation is the result of the stool traveling too slowly. Adding in more fiber and drinking more water, and exercise often helps.

If not, it may be a signal to other problems.

Diarrhea, on the other hand, is a result of the stool passing too quickly, especially through the large intestine where much of the water gets absorbed. This can result from stomach viruses, food allergies, intolerances, digestive disturbances amongst other things.

Either way, chronic constipation or diarrhea is not normal.

Listen to your body and pay attention to what it is telling you.

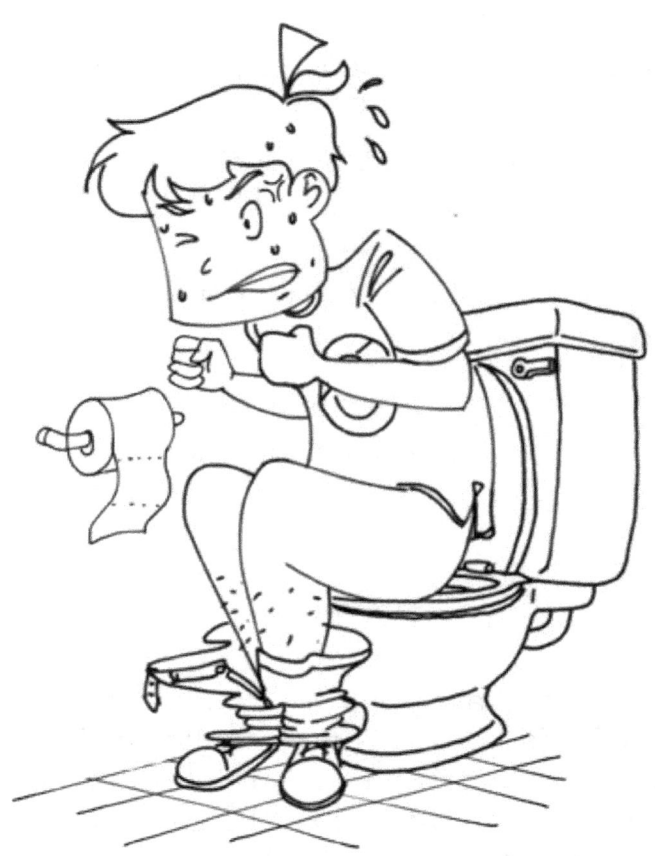

CHAPTER 7

Healthy Eating Manifesto
3 Day Detox

Looking to lighten up and get that body back into tiptop shape?

Do you suffer from any of these symptoms? It is a sign your body may need a Detox:

fatigue

resistance to weight loss

cravings

mental fog

sluggish elimination

mood swings

anxiety

immune issues

There are several types of detox diets. For the context of this book, I am referring to those detox diets which recommend consumption of foods that are essential for your health and beneficial to weight loss - organic foods, fruits and vegetables. This is done by cleansing out your body and improving your metabolism.

You can also do specialized cleanses designed specifically for a certain area of the body, for instance, the liver, kidneys, blood or lungs.

However, many detox programs just involve cleansing the entire body.

First of all, it is important that you have regular bowel movements during a detox because this will lessen the likelihood of toxins being reabsorbed by the body. A good way to make sure you will regularly eliminate is to take 2 tablespoons of ground flax seeds in lemon water in the morning, and drink lemon water throughout the day. Flax seeds provide the body with fiber, and lemon water has a slightly laxative effect.

It is also important to drink enough fluids on a cleanse. You should try to include at least 8 glasses of water daily to ensure that you are allowing toxins to be flushed out.

As with any major change in your life, it is generally easier to accomplish your goals when you have the help and support of friends and family. Make a point to inform those close to you what you hope to accomplish. In addition, it's always a good idea to let them know exactly what you're doing, so they do not unintentionally sabotage your plans. Perhaps, they will even want to join you. The presence of a buddy who can keep you on track and motivated will significantly decrease the chances that you will give up before accomplishing your goals.

Read on for a sample of my 3-day detox diet that will satisfy anyone. Especially, if you are new to the world of detox diets, you'll love this.

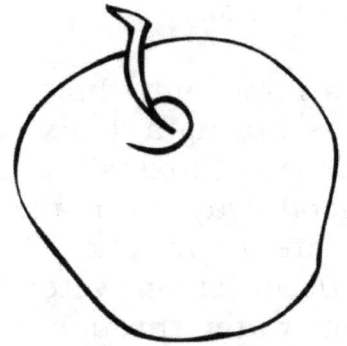

3 Day Healthy Eating Manifesto Detox

	BREAKFAST	LUNCH	DINNER	SNACKS (2x day)
DAY 1	Choice of Smoothie	Build your own salad	Vegetable broth Curried Lentils on Quinoa	Kale chips, small apple with pat of almond butter
DAY 2	Choice of Smoothie	Build your own salad	Zucchini & Eggplant Stew	Trail Mix, veggie sticks with hummus
DAY 3	Choice of Smoothie	Build your own salad	Lettuce Wraps	1/4 Cup raw almonds or walnuts, Baked apple or pear

NOTE: Chart your water intake. Aim for (8)-8 oz. glasses daily.

This detox honors those who are also vegans as meat is only an option during lunch as an add-on.

UPON RISING:
1/2 lemon squeezed into a glass of warm water
MID-DAY:
1 tablespoon of bentonite clay and 1 tablespoon of ground flaxseeds in a glass of water

Breakfast Smoothies:

Choice 1:	Choice 2:	Choice 3:
1 c coconut water	1 c almond milk	1/2 c almond milk
1/2 avocado	1/2 banana	1 1/2 Tbsp. almond butter
1/2 c strawberries	1/2 c strawberries	1 TBS honey
1/4 c blueberries	1/2 c frozen pineapple slices	1/2 TBS cacao
1c baby spinach	1c baby spinach	1 banana 1c ice cubes

Optional Add-ons: protein powder (plant based protein only), chia seeds, flax or hemp seeds, spices and any other super foods. I often add in about an ounce of organic goji juice. ADD all ingredients to blender and enjoy!

Lunchtime: Build Your Own Salad
Pick your salad: arugula, spinach, spring mix, romaine
Add some more greens: cucumbers, broccoli, avocado, sprouts
Add a bit of color: tomato, red onion, shredded carrots, radish, cranberry, artichoke
Add some crunch: apple, pear, seeds, and nuts
Protein Power Up: grilled chicken, grilled fish, garbanzo beans, lentils
Dress it up: balsamic vinaigrette, oil & vinegar

Snacks

Kale Chips
Preheat oven to 375°
Organic Kale (I recommend Trader Joe's)
1 TBS olive oil
Sprinkle of Celtic or Pink Himalayan Sea Salt
Dash of Pepper (optional)

Place on baking sheet or baking stone.
Bake approximately 15 minutes or until edges browned.

Trail Mix	Baked Apple or Pear (preheat oven to 350°)
almonds	Core apple or pear & add in cinnamon
sunflower seeds	nutmeg, spices, few raisins
unsweetened raisins	Bake approx. 20-25 minutes.
Just mix equal parts together.	

Dinner

Zucchini and Eggplant Stew
This recipe will actually make 3 reasonable sized portions. If you are eating it alone, then freeze two portions, just to eat within the next few days, or even at the end of your detox, as a healthy alternative. (Maybe even extend your detox a day or 2.)
- 1 onion, chopped
- 1 zucchini, cut into chunks
- 1 eggplant, cut into 1" cubes
- 1 can peeled tomatoes (no sugar or salt added)
- 4 finely chopped tomatoes
- Fresh basil

Lightly stir fry the onion in ½ teaspoon of extra virgin olive oil. Add the zucchini and eggplant. After a couple of minutes add the chopped tomatoes and the can of tomatoes, along with a little fresh basil. Bring to a boil, and then let it simmer for about 20 minutes or so. Before serving, add in the rest of the fresh basil and enjoy.

Curried Lentils over Quinoa
4 servings

- 1/2 cup dried lentils
- 1 cup water
- 3/4 cup coconut milk
- 1 tsp. curry powder
- sea salt to taste
- 1 cup prepared quinoa

Prepare quinoa according to directions or prepare in advance and refrigerate.
Rinse lentils and place in a saucepan with the water. Bring to a boil and simmer over low heat for 15 minutes. Stir in the curry powder, coconut milk and season with salt to taste. Return to a simmer, and cook for an additional 10 to 15 minutes, until tender. Serve over quinoa.

Homemade Vegetable Broth
Active time: 15 minutes Total time: 4 hours
Makes about 1 gallon.

Approx. 6 cups of chopped veggies. Consider using carrots, onion, tomato, parsnip, basil etc.
1 bunch of parsley
1 gallon water
A large pot with a lid

In a pot, add water and veggies (except the parsley), and bring to a boil. Then reduce to a simmer and leave covered on the stovetop for about 4 hours.
Approximately, 30 minutes before it's done, toss

in the parsley and finish cooking.

Then, strain it into some mason jars. Set them in the refrigerator to cool. Put in ice cube trays for quick use. Keeps in the fridge for a few days, and indefinitely in the freezer.

Lettuce Wraps

This makes for an attractive appetizer at a party, or just for the heck of it!

- 2 ripe avocados, pitted and mashed
- 2 tomatoes, chopped
- ½ yellow onion, diced
- 2 cloves fresh garlic, chopped
- ¼ cup fresh chopped parsley
- organic corn (cooked)
- Juice from half a lime
- 6-8 romaine lettuce leaves (large)

Add the first seven ingredients to a large medium bowl. Mix until well combined. Place two tablespoons of the mixture in the center of each lettuce leaf. Roll the leaf up and present it on a platter.

What to do throughout the day?

Sip plenty of herbal teas. Drink plenty of water with some fresh squeezed lemon, it is alkalizing and gets the lymphatic's flowing. Aim to drink at least 4 pints of fluid a day.

Keep a journal of how you feel and the ways in which your body seems to be reacting. This can be helpful to learn lessons from your detox so that you can adapt a generally healthier lifestyle after your program has ended.

- Listen to your body. You are going to try new food and new mind/body exercises this week. After each, pay attention to how your body feels. Notice if you have more/less energy. Pay attention to your digestion and see what food flavors your body likes or fights. This week is about finally taking the time to tune into your body's needs.

- Adjust exercise routine. Take longer walks outside and do some yoga. Your body will be using some of that external exercise energy to rebuild and repair internally. Yoga and walking are still great for that exercise burn, getting the blood flowing and elimination system flushing. Keep taking medications. If you are on any prescribed medications by a licensed health care professional, please continue taking them. Please let them know what you are doing and seek their approval, if appropriate.

Take a mini-mental vacation from work. If you experience stress or unbalance with your current work situation, take this one week to leave work at work. No need to actually take the time off. This is about allowing your mind and body to have your full personal attention to jump-start its healing. Hanging onto excess stress, both physically and mentally, will not allow you to flourish.

What to do when things feel bad

Some people who have been on a detox program will tell you that it was so easy, they just sailed through, they never even thought about burgers, fries or a glass of wine. No, they just had a great week or 10 days, and all they ate was a spinach leaf (ok, that was an exaggeration, but you get the picture, don't you?). Others will tell you that it was bad. Really bad. They spent a whole week or 10 days dreaming about burgers, fries, wine, beer and so on. It was hell. They thought they would crack up and so on and so on.

So which experience will you have? Well to some extent that depends on your mindset. If you think that you will enjoy it and you know that you have lots of little tricks up your sleeve, to make the process as easy as possible, then you probably will go through it without any real difficulties. But there may be times when you may find that it feels a little bit harder than others: a stressful day, the kids are misbehaving, or work just has been real tough. Well, when this happens, then you need to bring out the 'Big guns' and these are the tricks that will simply calm you back down and help you become more focused again.

YOGA/STRETCHES

If you have never done yoga, now may be a good time to start. Enroll in a beginner's class. If you have done it before, then go along to a class and just refresh yourself with the techniques. If you can't face a class or begin something new, then simply stretch your body as much as you can. Stretch upwards, lifting your arms to the ceiling, breathing inwards deeply, and then bend down towards the floor, keeping your arms and legs straight, exhale as you do this. Keep your breathing steady and even. Try to do this every time you feel stressed or uptight. If you are at work, go to the restroom and do it in private. At home, you can do it anywhere that is quiet and peaceful.

EXERCISE

Exercise will help relax your body as well as releasing toxins, so it is important to keep up the exercise and not let things slide: remember this is an important part of the overall program.

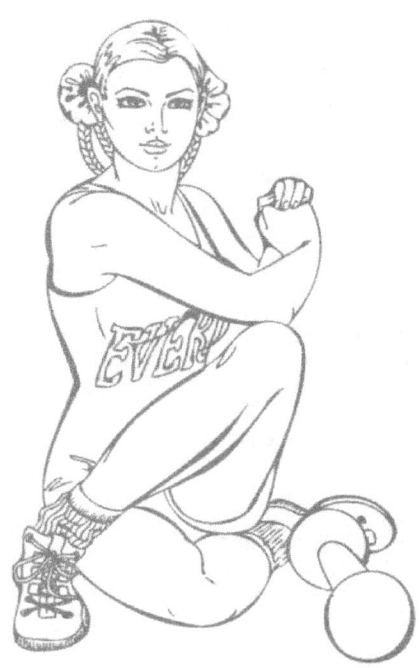

DEEP BREATH

Deep breathing really does calm the body down. This is a scientific fact, so use it to ensure that you keep your body and soul calm and composed. Breathe in slowly, through your nose, to a count of 8. Hold the breath there for a count of 6. Then breathe out again, to a count of 10. Yes, you are breathing out for longer than you are breathing in, but this is what actually calms you down the fastest. Some people advise deep breathing once an hour, for at least the first few days of a detox program, but it is up to you. You can either do it as often as once an hour or you can just do it whenever you feel yourself becoming a little bit stressed. Just like sweating is detoxifying to the skin, deep breathing is detoxifying to the lungs.

AROMATHERAPY

Have a few drops of lavender in a relaxing bath, or buy some good quality almond oil and mix in a few drops of your favorite relaxing aromatherapy oil. Then apply whenever you feel anxious or uptight. If you apply it to your pulse points, then you can breathe it in and this will actually help you to calm down much quicker.

PATTERNS OF THOUGHT

We are what we think to a large extent, which means that we are capable of effecting change, even when we may not be aware of this power. Often if we have been living a toxic lifestyle, then our patterns of thought are also pretty toxic. If we are always thinking negatively or focusing on bad stuff, rather than being gentle with ourselves and thinking positive thoughts, about how well we are doing, how much love there is in our lives and so on. All these negative thoughts need to be fought. Try to repeat affirmations to yourself on a regular basis throughout the detox program and change your 'toxic thoughts' into sweet, life-affirming ones. This can take some time to get used to, but it really does work, so make an effort to think positively and in an upbeat fashion.

End of Detox

Now that you have reached the end of the detox, what do you do? Do you crack open a bottle of wine; sit down to burgers and fries and then several candy bars? Well, if you do, then you probably are going to find that you need to detox again pretty soon. Try to learn from your detox and make sure that you reduce the amount of processed food, sweet, sugary food, caffeine and alcohol that you consume on a regular basis and steer clear of the salt cellar.

A detox program such as this can help you make long-term changes to your diet and ensure that you lead a happier life, with less stress and fatigue. Your intestines, kidneys, skin, bowel, liver and even your brain will be given good food with all the nutrients that your body needs, without having to deal with toxins or poisons that you consume regularly.

Your body is now cleansed, so try to keep it that way and ensure that your body is maintained at its optimum state of health and fitness. If you do this, then you will also find that next time you detox it is a much easier process to go through.

Healthy Eating Manifesto
~ Shopping List for *LIFE* ~

PRODUCE

apples
apricot
artichoke
arugula
asparagus
avocado
banana
beets
bell peppers
blackberries
blueberries
bok choy
broccoli
broccoli rabe
butternut squash
cabbage
cantaloupe
carrots
cauliflower
celery
cherries
coconut
collard greens
cranberries
cucumber
eggplant
figs
grapes
grapefruit
green beans
goji berries
jicama
kale
kiwi
leeks
lemon
lettuces
lime
mango
mushrooms
nectarine
okra
onion
oranges
papaya
peas
peaches
pears
peppers
pineapple
plums
pomegranate
pumpkin
radish
rhubarb
sea vegetables
spinach
squash
sweet potato
swiss chard
tomatoes

turnip
watercress
watermelon

tuna
Avoid shellfish
& mollusks

MEAT
(grass-fed,
organic)
beef, lean
bison
chicken
eggs
lamb
turkey
venison
wild game
No pork

DAIRY
(organic,
limited
amounts)
clarified butter
Greek yogurt
kefir
goat cheese
unprocessed cheese

SEAFOOD
(Wild only)
(cold water
sources are best)
bass
cod
flounder
grouper
haddock
halibut
herring
mackerel
mahi mahi
snapper
salmon
sardines
trout

NUTS & SEEDS
(raw/not roasted)
almonds
brazil
buckwheat
cashew
chia
flax
hemp
hazelnuts
macadamia
millet
pecans
pine
pistachio
pumpkin
quinoa
sesame
sunflower
walnuts

almond butter
nut butters
No peanuts

OILS
almond
coconut
grapeseed
extra virgin olive
sesame
walnut
No canola

SPICES & HERBS
basil
black pepper
cayenne
chili pepper
cilantro
cinnamon
cloves
cumin
curry
dill
fennel
garlic
ginger
mint
nutmeg
oregano
paprika
parsley
rosemary
sage

tarragon
thyme
turmeric

BEVERAGES
almond milk,
unsweetened
coconut milk
coconut water
coffee (organic)
herbal teas
kombucha
roobios tea
vegetable juice (raw)
water (filtered)

SWEET STUFF
(limit)
agave (organic)
cacao
dark chocolate
maple syrup/yacon
(pure, organic)
raw honey
stevia

CONDIMENTS
apple cider vinegar
balsamic vinegar
Bragg's aminos
ketchup (organic)
mustard (organic)
mayo (organic)
salsa

salt (pink Himalayan
or quality sea salt)
tamari

MISC
brown rice
black rice
mung beans

Good Eating Habits

Most everyone knows that good eating habits are essential to good health and well-being. While many people seem to ignore this fact, lots of people really do try to eat properly. Part of the problem is that many people don't seem to be able to maintain good eating habits is both misinformation as well as lack of information.

With the vast variety of foods out there and the huge amount of advertising done, (often with misleading statements), it would stand to reason that it is so easy to be guided off track and right into bad food choice territory. Add to the equation the enormous amount of diet plans for weight loss, as well as the amount of trendy new cookbooks extolling the virtues of the latest fad healthy foods to eat, and you have a tremendous array of contradicting information coming at you from all sides!

So what should you do to develop good eating habits? Here are some guidelines to follow to get you well on your way to making better, more health minded food choices.

1) PREPARE YOURSELF FOR SUCCESS
 In order to begin you need to prepare yourself mentally. Plan in advance what you will be eating during the week, write it out for yourself, stock up on those foods and make it happen.

2) PROTEIN IS VITAL
 Make sure you eat protein in some form at almost every meal.

3)   ELIMINATE OR EAT LESS REFINED BREADS AND STARCHES

Cut back on the amount of bread and pasta you consume. If you must, eat your pasta as your mid-day meal and make it organic and gluten-free. If you do eat bread, good sources are freshly made sourdough (due to the fermentation process) or fresh millet bread (gluten-free).

Check your local health food stores to steer you in the right direction.

Confession: I grew up on bread and pasta. I rarely touch it anymore.
Why? My belly thanks me for it and I feel so much better.

4)   LIMIT YOUR DAIRY CONSUMPTION

Substitute almond milk or rice or coconut milk. Low-fat yogurt has a very high sugar content, go for the organic plain yogurt and add in your own fresh fruit.

5)   DON'T OVERDO THE FRUIT

No more than 2 a day and use just the good fiber kinds. Apples, pears, plums, and berries are best. Totally avoid fruit juices; they're loaded with sugar.

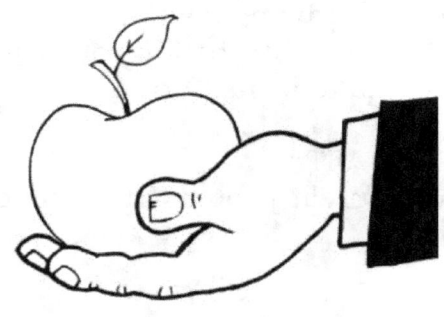

6)   EAT NUTS
    Just stay in moderation here. A quarter cup of pistachios, almonds or cashews are not only tasty, but a good source of protein.

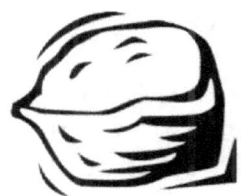

7)   REDUCE THE PORTIONS
    When at home, use smaller plates. If you go out, order the smaller size or if one size fits all, get a doggie bag in advance and put half your meal in it before you start to eat. You will feel better and have a good meal to eat again later.
If you make good choices, you will have plenty of food to eat, so portion shouldn't be a major issue.

8)   DRINK LOTS OF WATER
Water has great dietary and overall health benefits. Many hunger pangs are due to lack of water. Drinking plenty of water throughout the day will keep you hydrated and will reduce food cravings.

9)   GO MEATLESS FOR AT LEAST 1 DAY/WEEK
    Try eating at least one day with no meat.

10)   NEVER SKIP BREAKFAST
Breakfast gets your metabolism going. Make yourself a great smoothie that packs a punch and keeps you satiated.

11) EAT MORE SEAFOOD

Eat water packed tuna and salmon; they are loaded with omega-3 fatty acids that help protect the heart. You should have this seafood 2-3 times per week. Check for mercury content. Cold water, wild sources of seafood are often the best choice.

12) BRING YOUR OWN LUNCH

Rather than eating lunch out all of the time, make your lunch and only eat out for lunch once a week. You will save money and know your eating good things like lean chicken and fruit or veggies.

The fact is if you use these simple guidelines as a means to put together a plan of good eating habits you will be well on your way to developing them with sound nutrition and you will be paving the way for a life-long journey of better health.

CHAPTER 8

ANY RESERVATIONS?

Eating Out? But of course!

Dreaming of your favorite Italian restaurant?

Do you fancy French?

Indulge in Indian?

Chomp on Chinese?

Whatever you choose the options can be dizzying.

As with anything in life there are good choices and not so good choices.

With tempting menus, large portions, and a festive atmosphere, it's easy to skip healthy eating.

It's okay to splurge every now and then, although you'll pack on the weight if you make it a habit.

When you eat out at restaurants, always be smart about it.

I am happy to say, as a serial restaurant frequenter; most dining establishments are very accommodating to your dietary needs.

With so many people these days becoming more aware, restaurants are starting to take notice.

For example, many restaurants now offer many gluten-free options, which I am so happy about. If you have any allergies or lactose intolerance issues, just let them know. Most restaurants are happy to accommodate your needs. All you have to do is ... Speak Up ... (Politely, of course)

If you are on a low-sodium diet, tell them to skip the salt. I bring my own pink Himalayan sea salt with me, so I'm in control of how much goes in and it's a healthier alternative to processed table salt.

Request that your food is prepared with very little or no butter or better yet, ask if they can use just a tad bit of olive oil instead.

CHAPTER 9

WAISTLINE or WASTE LINE?

If you eat right and exercise, you will have a waistline.

If you don't, it will be a waste line, don't let that happen to you.

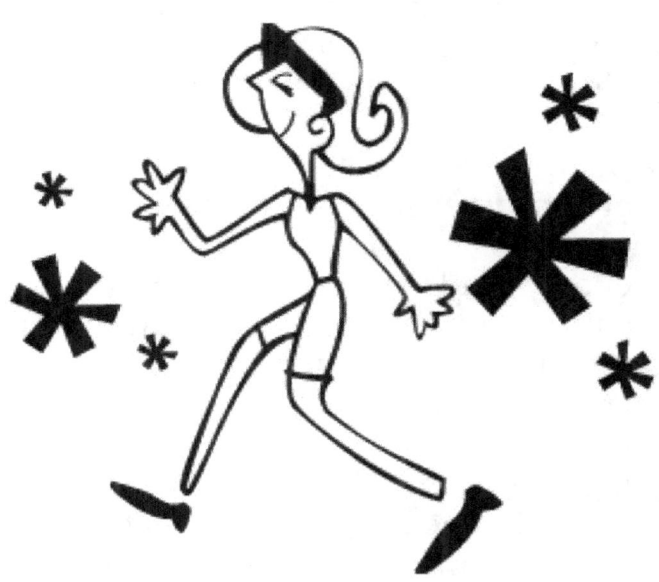

There are 4 basic categories of physical activity or exercise:

This includes aerobic, strength, balance and flexibility. Mixing up your routine is your best bet as it reduces boredom, and each one concentrates on different things.

1) Aerobic activity increases your heart rate and makes your heart more efficient. It focuses on continuous movement especially with your large muscle groups. It can range from low to high levels of intensity. Examples of aerobic activity include: brisk walking, jogging, cycling, dancing and swimming.

2) Strength exercises make your muscles stronger. Even small increases in strength can make a big difference. Maintaining strength and muscle mass is extremely important for healthy aging. Lifting weights or use of resistance bands are some forms of strength training.

3) Balance or stability exercises improve the body's alignment. Another great thing about stability training is all the work to hold your balance requires extra attention from your core. When you work on an unstable surface, your muscles need to work harder to maintain your balance, resulting in increased muscle activity. Some examples include the use of a stability ball, planks, squats and lunges.

114

4) <u>Flexibility</u> enhances the range of motion of your muscles and joints to move to their full range of motion. It stretches your muscles so your body can stay lean and limber. Yoga and Pilates are excellent ways to stay flexible.

Some fun things to consider to keep you *moving*:

- Zumba - great aerobic workout if you love to dance.
- Belly Dancing - works your core, dance and have fun all at once.
- Yoga - so many different kinds: check out what is right for you.
- Pilates - strengthens the core and makes you feel so flexible.
- Cardio/Aerobic – raises heart rate (our bodies were meant to move) recommended 3x per week.
- Free-Weights - builds bone mass and muscle 2-3x/week.
- Rebounding - great for circulation and lymphatic system 1-2x/week.

So what moves you?

Find an activity that makes you happy and get your body in action.

> Remember it's important to move your body daily. Even on a super-busy day, find some creative ways to add in some movement. Take a walk outdoors, go for a swim or simply dance around the house. Park your car at the far end of the lot. You will increase your circulation, feel better and change your thoughts.

"Walking is man's best medicine."
~ Hippocrates

Inspiring Tips for Looking Great and Feeling Slimmer

Dress for your Body type.

This is a biggie. Have you ever noticed someone walk by and in the back of your mind wondered if they owned a mirror? Don't fall victim to what I refer to as a "fashion faux-pas."
You certainly don't need to be a fashionista all of the time, but let's face it, the options for looking fabulous are limitless.
Experiment with your wardrobe and make a party out of it on a rainy day. Invite a friend over whose opinion you trust and will help you sort out the good stuff from the not-so-good stuff.
What you are looking for is an honest evaluation of what fits and what doesn't fit.
Out of what does fit, go through all the things that you like.

Dress for your age range.

Another biggie. If your 62 and dress like a 22-year-old, it doesn't work. You have to pass the torch already. It doesn't matter how great you may look, find clothes that are more mature and enhance your assets.

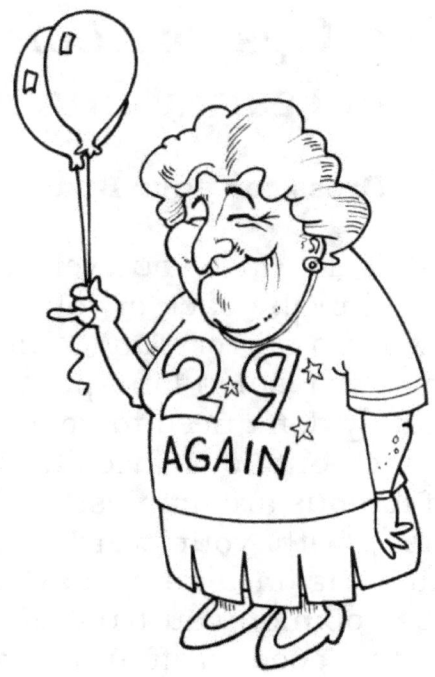

TIP: Keep only clothes that *fit* in your closet and clothes that you *like*. Trust me. It is an absolute pleasure to walk into your closet and know you can just pick something off the hanger that is just perfect.

What a time-saver, instead of fumbling through "oh, only if I lost 5 more pounds."

I admit; it is difficult to part with clothes that you like and that almost fit. Find a separate closet and put them in there.

When you reach your goal, you can go "shop" in that closet all over again.

I've done this myself with great success. I made a major move from New York to Florida, and I donated about 75% of my clothing.

It felt so freeing. Sometimes less is more.
I did hold on to my "better clothes", one's that I had a few pounds to lose to make them a part of my everyday wardrobe. Once, I got settled in, and shed a few, I was over the moon. Those bit too tight clothes were now looking good. Yes, right back into the big closet. Then cleared the stuff in the big closet that was now too big. Again, I only save a few of the best and pricey items, so I don't need to juggle too much.

MAKE IT FUN

DECLUTTER - Keep your Closet Organized.
You will thank me.

POSTURE
Stand tall and proud
Shoulders back
Belly pulled in
Butt out
Smile (attitude means a lot)

You will look taller, thinner, be more approachable and feel more confident!

"Work like you don't need the money, love like your heart has never been broken, and dance like no one is watching."
                    ~Aurora Greenway

CHAPTER 10

SKIN DEEP

We've all heard the expression "you are what you eat," and your skin is no exception.

Simple Fact: Your skin is your largest organ. It is our protective covering and our first line of defense to fight illness and disease. It is also a passageway to our bloodstream. That being said, what you apply topically on your skin as well as what you eat will affect the overall health and appearance of your skin.

LET'S GET STARTED FROM THE INSIDE OUT.

A quote from one of my favorite skin docs:

"Certain foods have powerhouse ingredients that keep skin supple and smooth and help fight age-related damage," says Nicholas Perricone, MD, a board-certified dermatologist and author of Ageless Face, Ageless Mind.

First, we need to hydrate the skin. That means drinking plenty of water, at least the recommended 6-8 glasses per day. If you are physically active, live in a warm-climate or feel thirsty you may need to up your daily intake.

As we age, skin tends to become dehydrated much quicker (causing wrinkles), so ample hydration is key.

Eat your Super-Foods. If it's good for your health, it's good for your skin too.

SOME EXAMPLES:

Omega 3 Fatty Acids-found in fatty fish, such as herring, sardines and salmon. Other sources of Omega 3's include flaxseeds and walnuts. Omega 3's are known to decrease inflammation, and may reduce the risk of acne and other skin problems.

Vitamin C produces collagen and prevents cells from damage caused by free radicals. Great sources are oranges, pineapples, tomato, strawberries and bell peppers.

Vitamin E helps limit sun damage and signs of aging. Almonds are a terrific source of Vitamin E.

Vitamin A revitalizes skin by increasing cell production and rebuilds tissue. Eggs and dark leafy greens are good choices.

Beta-Carotene needed for growth and repair of tissue. Think orange foods, carrots, sweet potato, pumpkin, and cantaloupe.

Other fabulous foods to include boosting your skin health: dark leafy vegetables, avocados, mushrooms, berries and surprise, dark chocolate!

Did you know that your skin is a "breathable" organ?

Up to 60% of what you apply topically on your skin will be absorbed into your bloodstream and children absorb even more than that.

Imagine products you've been using for years actually contain harmful ingredients and could damage your health. Your first instinct should be to find a healthier alternative - pronto!

Heightened awareness and potential dangers have caused consumers to take a closer look at what they put on their skin and demand safer alternatives.

Many cosmetic companies do **not** list their ingredients aka "toxic" chemicals because they are not required to do so.

Several of these toxic chemicals are linked to a host of problems including allergies, skin rashes, cancer, headaches, fertility and reproductive issues, birth defects, hormone inhibitors and more.

Some toxic chemicals that should be avoided:

Parabens - often found in deodorants and moisturizers... a hormone inhibitor and believed to accelerate tumor growth.

Phthalates - are used in cosmetics and personal care products, including perfume, hair spray, soap, shampoo, nail polish, and skin moisturizers. They are also used in many other consumer products such as flexible plastic and vinyl toys, shower curtains, wallpaper, food packaging, and plastic wrap. Phthalates are hormone disruptors in the body and are linked to abdominal obesity and insulin resistance.

Artificial fragrance/color - may trigger allergies, or asthma. Some colors contain lead and harmful dyes.

Toluene - found in nail polish, hair-color products and some fragrances. Linked to kidney and liver damage, may affect fetal growth.

Sodium Lauryl Sulfate /Sodium Laureth Sulfate - a foaming agent found in shampoos, body/facial washes. Dries out the skin and linked to eczema, hair-loss, rashes, dry, scaly skin.

Formaldehyde - is known by several different names and should be avoided at all costs. Side effects are numerous.

PEG's - this is anti-freeze. Use it for your car, not your skin. Is used in numerous skin and personal care products.

Paraffin/Mineral Oil/Petrolatum - clogs pores = toxic build-up. Phthalates are found in plastics. It is a known hormone disruptor. Triclosan is used in anti-bacterial products. It is a pesticide and harmful to the environment. It is also a suspected carcinogenic.

Sunscreens - just Google some of those ingredients. Possible damage to DNA and many are known carcinogens.

There are over 1800 products on the market to choose from, making it incredibly confusing and difficult to pick the best and safest brand. Here's what you need to watch out for:

- Oxybenzone - this is a hormone-disrupting chemical which penetrates the skin and enters the bloodstream. It is the most popular ingredient in chemical based sunscreens and only blocks UVB ray (sun's good rays that provide vitamin D production), not UVA which are the most free radical damaging rays. Avoid any sunscreen that has this chemical at all costs, especially for children.
- Vitamin A (Retinyl Palmitate) – A 2009 study by U.S. government scientists released by the National Toxicology Program found when this is applied to the skin in the presence of sunlight, it may speed the development of skin tumors and lesions.
- Fragrance – Sure it may make the product smell nice, but this is a petroleum based product linked to organ toxicity and allergies.

- High SPF (Sun Protection Factor) – The FDA does not regulate SPF higher than 50, and there's no scientific proof they work better than lower SPF. Many of the higher SPFs do not provide any additional protection, and studies have suggested users are exposed to as many or more ultraviolet rays as those who use lower SPF products.
- Sprays or Powders – Generally speaking, sprays and powders have additional chemicals added to them for performance purposes. These additional chemicals are, usually, not something you want to be spraying on your body and can be toxic to the lungs. Besides, remember sunscreen is formulated for your skin, not your lungs. Many of the side effects of sprays and powders on the lungs are not tested before being approved.
- Popular Conventional Brands – Beware, even your beloved favorites (I won't name them here) are rated the worst in terms of safety in the Environmental Working Group's Sunscreen Guide. You can use this guide to find out how good or bad the brand you have or want to buy is rated. Please do this!

Choosing A Safe Sunscreen:

Look for titanium dioxide and zinc oxide-based mineral sunscreens, which do not penetrate the skin and provide UVA protection against the sun's most damaging rays.

- Use non-nano products that do not have small particles that can absorb into the skin.
- Use sunscreens that are unscented or use essential oils as fragrance.
- Look for a lotion-based sunscreen with water resistance.
- Choose broad-spectrum sunscreens that protect against UVA and UVB rays.

Choose sunscreen products that are rated 0-2 in the Environmental Working Group's Sunscreen Guide. If it's a toxin; it doesn't belong on your skin.

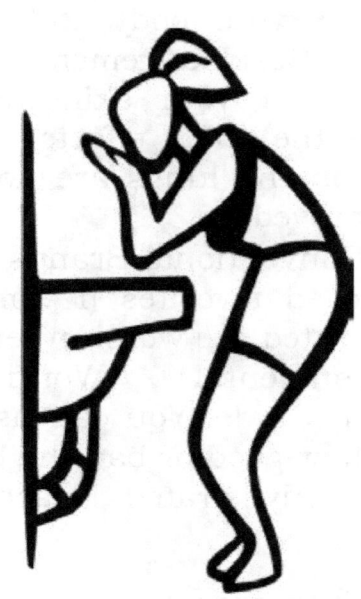

CHAPTER 11

LOVE and CHANGE YOUR LIFE

Positive Thoughts and the Power of Intention: Keeping Yourself Healthy Through Positive Thinking

So you're having a fight with your partner. You can no longer stand to be around your best friend. This day is just destroying your life. Struggles with moods, depression and anxiety, are obstacles felt by everyone, but they shouldn't rule your life. Take some time out of your day to help yourself feel better and to strengthen your well-being through positive thought.

Keep in mind that you cannot fix the people around you, and trying can be like slamming your head against a brick wall. Instead, if you're having problems with others, always take an intrinsic look at yourself. You're the one responsible for your well-being. With time, devotion to feeling good and a sense of positive energy, you can step away from negative situations and put yourself in a position of greater peace.

Some situations cannot be fixed. It's frustrating when you want so badly for something to work itself out, at work, in friendship, on a sports team, but consider it might just not be meant to be. Think about the reasons you are trying at something. Is it to make you happy, or to impress others and fulfill a commitment? You don't owe anyone your happiness. Take control of your life by removing yourself from situations and environments that are poorly affecting your mood and ability to be positive towards yourself and those around you.

Take a break. Recuperate. Think of living life the same way as you'd take a test. If you keep coming at a problem over and over again it will start making less and less sense, and you'll become more and more frustrated and burnt out. It's the same way with life. Our bodies and our minds require rejuvenation. Take that mental health day off from work. Hire a babysitter or a pet sitter for the evening, and take a moment out for yourself. Take a hot bath. Meditate. Eat a fabulous meal that you didn't have to cook. Pray. Do something you've wanted to do forever, or take a little trip to reward yourself for just living.

Remember you deserve to be on this planet. Even when you're not thinking about it, your good, strong body is breathing for you. You're here for a reason. Stop beating yourself up with guilt and regret, these are just bags that weigh you down when you should be moving on to the next part of your life. Make some lists of goals for yourself, and achievable objectives to reach these goals. Having a plan can take away the stress of that nagging responsibility to be "doing something." Make a list of all your strengths, specific ones, and read them to yourself every once in a while (force yourself to read them even if you don't feel interested or deserving). This is not to make you feel "better," this is to help you recognize the person you are in all your goodness.

Feed yourself well. Just because you're a mom doesn't mean you have to eat leftover chicken nuggets. Just because you're a student on the run doesn't mean you have to eat fast food. Just because you're broke doesn't mean you don't have access to farmer's markets and healthy eating. You are a human; you are important; you are worth the effort and expense of vibrant health. Don't take yourself for granted. Nourish your body the way you want your soul to be nourished. Eat with friends, drink, laugh, talk. Enjoy your life through the good things your body takes in.

Assignment:
Write a Love Letter to Yourself.
- Focus on all the good you bring into the world
- Let go of the negative thoughts and limiting beliefs that are holding you back
- Focus on the positive
- Go easy on yourself

Even if you're having a super-busy day, take a few moments to nurture yourself.

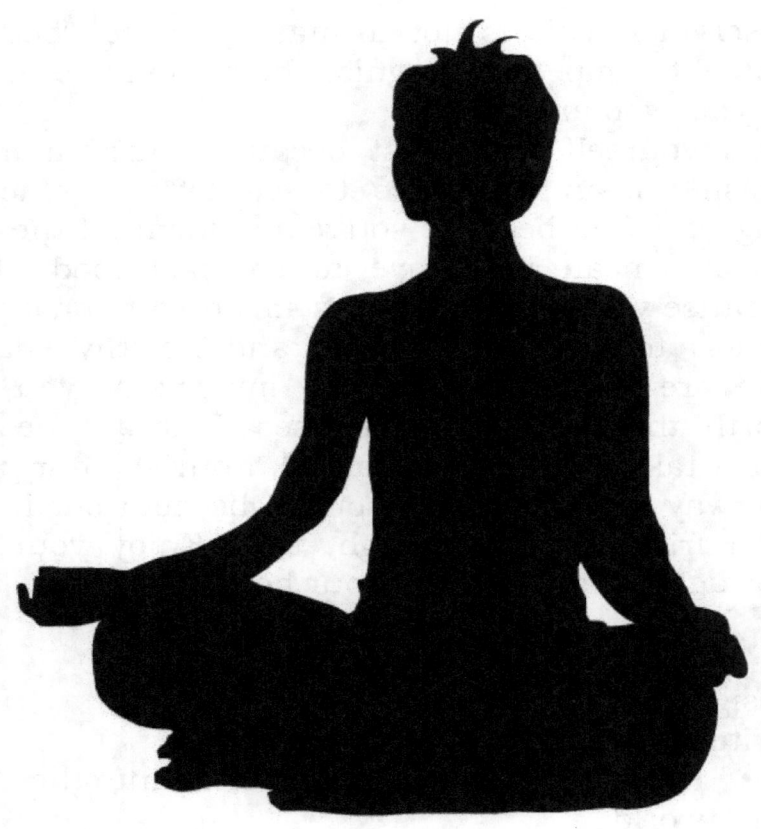

I call these little snippets of time "Peace Pockets."
Take a deep breathe in and repeat: "I am worthy –
let love be my inner guide."
Breathe out: resentment, fear – Repeat: "I am open
to giving and receiving love."

*Say, "yes" to challenges and dare to make
those big, bold dreams come true.
~Jacqueline Schiff*

CHANGE FOR LIFE

Change your patterns of thinking and adopt a lifestyle that is all about keeping your body cherished and nurtured. You clean your house and service your automobile, so why not your body? Make a conscious effort to think about the foods that you consume. Are they healthy, why are you eating them? If you are comfort eating or eating because you are stressed, in a rush or think that you don't have time to create a healthy and nutritious meal, then try to make the lifestyle changes that will enable you to have time to cherish and look after yourself.

This may take time, but, on the other hand, you are capable of taking active measures to rid your body of all the nastiness that has built up over the years, be it food or thought. Maintain the level of cleansing that you have achieved by eating a balanced and nutritious diet and within a month or so you will find that sweet, sugary foods or even very salty, processed foods have simply lost most of their appeal and instead you simply feel more energized and you have vitality, enthusiasm and a lust for life that you never knew you had. You eventually won't want to go back to your old eating and lifestyle habits because you'll be addicted to feeling and looking great. In other words, your new habits will become a part of your life.
It's all about savouring your wellness.
So simply enjoy all these new sensations, emotions and your whole new way of being.

REFERENCES

Real Weight Loss Solutions | Weight Loss. (n.d.). Retrieved from http://www.weight-loss-final-steps.com/articles/real-weight-loss-solutions/

The Standard American Diet in 3 Simple Charts | Mother Jones. (n.d.). Retrieved from http://www.motherjones.com/tom-philpott/2014/01/standard-american-diet-sad-charts

Poverty in the United States - Debt.org. (n.d.). Retrieved from http://www.debt.org/faqs/americans-in-debt/poverty-united-states/

Calculate Your BMI - Standard BMI Calculator. (n.d.). Retrieved from http://www.nhlbi.nih.gov/health/educational/lose_wt/BMI/bmicalc.htm

Sleep Your Way To Better Health - blogspot.com. (n.d.). Retrieved from http://siim-sleepproblems.blogspot.com/2008/12/sleep-your-way-to-better-health.html

Snooze to Lose Pounds - Weight-Loss - BoxingScene. (n.d.). Retrieved from http://www.boxingscene.com/weight-loss/58949.php

Types of Water Filters - Palma Health. (n.d.). Retrieved from http://www.palmahealth.com/typesofwaterfilters.html

Water Filters. (n.d.). Retrieved from http://www.snwa.com/wq/taste_home_filters.html

Drinking Alcohol When You Have High Cholesterol. (n.d.). Retrieved from http://www.webmd.com/cholesterol-management/cholesterol-and-alcohol

Alcohol Equivalence - Potsdam. (n.d.). Retrieved from http://www2.potsdam.edu/alcohol/AlcoholEquivalence.html

Wine: How Much Is Good for You? - WebMD. (n.d.). Retrieved from http://www.webmd.com/food-recipes/features/wine-how-much-is-good-for-you

5 Tips for cleaning out your pantry - SheKnows. (n.d.). Retrieved from http://www.sheknows.com/home-and-gardening/articles/844665/5-tips-for-cleaning-out-your-pantry

Hidden Salt in Foods — Health Hub from Cleveland Clinic. (n.d.). Retrieved from http://health.clevelandclinic.org/2013/07/hidden-salt-in-foods/

HEALTHY EATING MANIFESTO

Foods You Don't Have to Buy Organic - Dr. Andrew Weil. (n.d.). Retrieved from
http://www.drweil.com/drw/u/ART02984/Foods-You-Dont-Have-to-Buy-
Organic.html?print=1

Color Me Healthy — Eating for a Rainbow of Benefits. (n.d.). Retrieved from
http://www.todaysdietitian.com/newarchives/110308p34.shtml

What COLOUR is your diet? - for the love of it... (n.d.). Retrieved from
http://www.fortheloveofit.org.nz/awesome-eats/what-colour-is-your-diet

Count Colors Not Calories! - HealthStatus. (n.d.). Retrieved from
http://www.healthstatus.com/health_blog/body-fat-calculator-2/count-colors-not-
calories/

A Rainbow On Your Plate by Dr. Anjana Maitra. (n.d.). Retrieved from
http://www.bolokids.com/index.cfm?md=Content&sd=Articles&ArticleID=1386

Colorize Your Plate! | Gerard E. Mullin, M.D. (n.d.). Retrieved from
http://www.huffingtonpost.com/gerard-e-mullin-md/nutrition-month_b_1427391.html

Eat the Rainbow: Why are the colours we eat important for our ... (n.d.). Retrieved from
http://www.eatandthink.co.uk/library/eat-the-rainbow

Food Label Decoding - Food Labels - Tricks and Traps. (n.d.). Retrieved from
http://www.freedieting.com/food_labels.htm

Gray Clinic offers food label tips. (n.d.). Retrieved from
http://weightloss.grayclinic.com/labels.html

Natural Body Detox Guide - What Are Toxins? (n.d.). Retrieved from
http://www.easyhomeremedy.com/Natural-Body-Detox-Guide/What-Are-Toxins.html

The Pros and Cons of a Body Detox | Rapid Body Detox. (n.d.). Retrieved from
http://rapidbodydetox.com/the-pros-and-cons-of-a-body-detox/

Detox Your Body in 10 Days. (n.d.). Retrieved from
http://download.inboxgeek.com/detox_in_10_days.pdf

7 Day Detox Diet Plan « Creating Vibrant Health with a Raw ... (n.d.). Retrieved from
http://rawfoodsolution.com/7-day-detox-diet-plan-529.html

Body Detox Guide - Natural Home Body Detox Program DAY 5. (n.d.). Retrieved from
http://www.easyhomeremedy.com/Natural-Body-Detox-Guide/Natural-Home-Body-
Detox-Program-DAY-5.html

Recipes : Go Local. (n.d.). Retrieved from

http://golocaldirect.com/article/art/Health/Raw-Food-Diet/130-Recipes.html

Body Detox Guide - Natural Home Body Detox Program DAY 1. (n.d.). Retrieved from http://www.easyhomeremedy.com/Natural-Body-Detox-Guide/Natural-Home-Body-Detox-Program-DAY-1.html

Body Detox Guide - What To Do When Things Feel Bad. (n.d.). Retrieved from http://www.easyhomeremedy.com/Natural-Body-Detox-Guide/What-To-Do-When-Things-Feel-Bad.html

Body Detox Guide - End Of Home Body Detox. (n.d.). Retrieved from http://www.easyhomeremedy.com/Natural-Body-Detox-Guide/End-Of-Home-body-Detox.html

Good Eating Habit - Walking Off The Weight. (n.d.). Retrieved from http://www.walkingofftheweight.com/articles/good-eating-habit.html

Curried Lentils Recipe - Allrecipes.com. (n.d.). Retrieved from http://allrecipes.com/Recipe/Curried-Lentils/

How to Eat Healthy While Travelling and Keep your Digestion ... (n.d.). Retrieved from http://www.patriciaeales.com/how-to-eat-healthy-while-travelling-and-keep-you/

Eating Healthy On The Run We-Help-All.com. (n.d.). Retrieved from http://we-help-all.com/wehelpall.com/eating-healthy-on-the-run/

10 great stability exercises for a strong core. (n.d.). Retrieved from http://www.king5.com/story/news/health/2014/08/03/13229598/

Loving Your Skin - Janelle Anderson — Working Site. (n.d.). Retrieved from http://janelleanderson.com/uncategorized/loving-your-skin/

The Ingredients In Sunscreen Are Destroying Your Health | RAW ... (n.d.). Retrieved from http://rawforbeauty.com/blog/the-ingredients-in-sunscreen-are-destroying-your-health.html

Body Detox Guide - End Of Home Body Detox. (n.d.). Retrieved from http://www.easyhomeremedy.com/Natural-Body-Detox-Guide/End-Of-Home-body-Detox.html

ABOUT

Linda Celauro, a leading expert in the field of Holistic Health and Weight Loss, has spent her career searching for the ideal lifestyle for optimal health and wellness. Linda obtained degrees in Psychology and Education from Hofstra University. She has obtained certifications as a Nutritional Consultant, Life Coach, Personal Trainer and Weight Loss Specialist. In 2012, Linda attended the Institute for Integrative Nutrition in New York, where she was trained in over 100 dietary theories, practical lifestyle management techniques, and innovative coaching methods with some of the world's top health and wellness experts.

Currently, Linda is a member of the International Association for Health Coaches and the American Association of Drugless Practitioners. She is regarded in her field as a Holistic Health expert.

Lindas passion for holistic medicine stems from her own life struggles and experiences. She spent many years of her life struggling on and off with IBS. Growing up, Linda coped with self-image issues as a kid that was a bit "chubby." Transitioning from her childhood to her teenage years, she became obsessed with food; she thought she was perfecting healthy eating but was really just eating all the wrong things "on the run

135

Throughout college, Linda tried to combat the IBS with pharmaceutical drugs, but none of them worked.

She realized it was time to take control of her life. Using food as medicine, Linda discovered not only the benefits of improved health, but the "secret" key to weight loss and maintenance.

Linda was born and raised in New York, but currently resides in southwest Florida with her husband. In her spare time, she enjoys boating, fine dining, and laughing with friends. Today, she continues to help clients reach their health and wellness goals. Linda offers in-person and online programs that include weight loss, fitness and clean-eating protocols.

Visit her on the web @ www.savourwellness.com

www.ingramcontent.com/pod-product-compliance
Lightning Source LLC
Chambersburg PA
CBHW070145290526
45789CB00002B/644